Applying the Results of Neuropsychological and Psychological Assessments

Neuropsychological and psychological evaluations in school settings are often rich in detail about a child's cognitive, academic, and emotional functions, and come with specific recommendations to support the child's performance in school. However, there is often a gap between the assessment results and the implementation of the recommendations, since learning specialists and teachers frequently do not have the means to both interpret and implement the recommendations. This manual presents clear and specific guidelines for school counselors and teachers to decode and put into practice evaluation findings.

The book begins by describing various functional domains that are assessed in a neuropsychological evaluation, and then notes how to recognize behavior and learning styles impacted by difficulty in one or more of the domains. Furthermore, it outlines activities that could be used in the classroom or other environments to support a child's weaknesses, develop new skills, or appeal to particular strengths. Finally, ready-to-use worksheets and activities are offered. This is an essential tool for school psychologists, special education teachers, and learning specialists and counselors.

Dawn E. Burau, LMHC, ATR and Sp.Ed, is core faculty at Lesley University in the Graduate School of Expressive Therapy. She has given multiple lectures at local and national conferences on topics related to special education, curriculum modification, use of arts in the school setting, and interpreting and applying neuropsychological assessments in the classroom and in the development of treatment plans. She worked as a teacher and therapist at the Community Therapeutic Day School for 13 years with children diagnosed with both learning disabilities and social/emotional disabilities.

Daniel K. Reinstein, Ph.D., is the Clinical Director and Director of Research at the Community Therapeutic Day School, where he has worked for the last thirty-six years. He also holds a faculty position in the Department of Psychiatry at the University of Massachusetts Medical School, where he teaches neuropsychology. He has been conducting Neuropsychological Evaluations over the last fifteen years.

Applying the Results of Neuropsychological and Psychological Assessments

A Manual for Teachers and Specialists

Dawn E. Burau and Daniel K. Reinstein

Routledge
Taylor & Francis Group
NEW YORK AND LONDON

First published 2018
by Routledge
711 Third Avenue, New York, NY 10017

and by Routledge
2 Park Square, Milton Park, Abingdon, Oxon, OX14 4RN

Routledge is an imprint of the Taylor & Francis Group, an informa business

Library of Congress Cataloguing-in-Publication Data
Names: Burau, Dawn E., author. | Reinstein, Daniel K., author.
Title: Applying the results of neuropsychological and psychological assessments : a manual for counselors and teachers / Dawn E. Burau and Daniel K. Reinstein.
Description: First edition. | New York : Routledge, [2018] | Includes index.
Identifiers: LCCN 2017026405| ISBN 9781138238879 (hbk) | ISBN 9781138238961 (pbk) | ISBN 9781315296333 (ebk)
Subjects: LCSH: Psychological tests for children. | Pediatric neuropsychology. | Problem children—Education.
Classification: LCC LB1131 .B829 2018 | DDC 371.94—dc23
LC record available at https://lccn.loc.gov/2017026405

ISBN: 978-1-138-23887-9 (hbk)
ISBN: 978-1-138-23896-1 (pbk)
ISBN: 978-1-315-29633-3 (ebk)

Typeset in Galliard
by Swales & Willis Ltd, Exeter, Devon, UK

To the families, colleagues and friends at CTDS who shared in our opportunity to learn, make mistakes, grow and write this manual.

Contents

Illustrations

Figure

Tables

Preface

In 2014, we published *Integrating Neuropsychological and Psychological Evaluations: Assessing and Helping the Whole Child* (Routledge), which argued that any comprehensive neuropsychological evaluation of a child should include not just tests of cognitive functioning, but also tests of emotional functioning in order to understand the "whole child's" needs. Since then, it has become increasingly clear that there is a significant gap between an assessment and its application in a school setting. This is largely due to the fact that teachers and specialists are overworked and overwhelmed by the amount of information they have to process about each of their students, let alone manage the added burden of applying the recommendations gleaned from an evaluation. To address this widening gap, we believed that a manual designed to facilitate the interpretation and implementation of results from a neuropsychological evaluation would be a timely and useful way to support both professionals and the students they strive to teach. *Applying the Results of Neuropsychological and Psychological Assessments: A Manual for Teachers and Specialists* is the outcome of that belief. We hope that it provides teachers and specialists with a very practical resource to not only more clearly understand neuropsychological data, but, more importantly, to translate that data into an understanding of a child's strengths and vulnerabilities. With this understanding, this manual can then act as a guide and provide specific suggestions for activities that will integrate results and interventions within a developmental and relationship-based context.

—Dawn E. Burau and Daniel K. Reinstein

Acknowledgments

Thank you to Nancy Fuller and Bruce Hauptman for their support and encouragement. Thank you, Perah Kessman, for your editing skills.

–1–

Implementing Evaluation Results in a School Setting

Introduction

It was getting to be too much. Leila had always been a difficult student, but by third grade her behaviors in the classroom were becoming intolerable to her teachers and peers in her small private school. She would talk non-stop, often interrupting anyone and everyone. When requested to do simple tasks within the classroom, she would often refuse with a simple, rude, "No." At times, she would lie across the top of her desk with feet, hands, and head dangling over the edge, and when asked to sit properly would oh-so-slowly peel herself off the desk and crawl back into her chair, where she would chew on the ends of her hair. In small group assignments, she would argue with peers if they didn't do things just right, or say hurtful things to her friends. She didn't seem to understand how the things she said could be hurtful; it was "just simple truth. I didn't mean to be mean." It all culminated when, while on an outing, she yelled "shut up" at her teacher and kicked her on the shin. These behaviors just didn't make sense because Leila was bright, very bright. She didn't struggle at all academically (with the exception that her handwriting was sloppy).

Teachers and friends were actually pretty accepting of Leila. She wasn't completely ostracized and the teachers felt Leila was likable. Leila could be kind, thoughtful, and funny. She had a way with words that was extremely clever. When she was engaged in a preferred activity, such as reading, she was extremely focused and self-reliant. Her drive for independence was admirable and she was a champion of the underdog. Despite her being so likable, the faculty were frustrated, having tried for years to really understand Leila's behavior and attitude, and they were beginning to think that maybe she was just mean, spoiled, and selfish. Maybe a different school was a better place for Leila.

At this point, school staff recommended to Leila's parents that she be assessed with a neuropsychological evaluation so they could better understand her needs. Leila was given a test

battery that assessed her cognitive strengths and vulnerabilities as well as her emotional state and social perceptions as a means to better understand her behavior.

With increasing regularity, school-aged children are being assessed and evaluated for various purposes. Screening occurs with the intent of identifying struggling students who may have a learning disability that could impact their ability to acquire academic skills. Assessment also occurs so that parents, clinicians, and teachers can better understand underlying factors associated with a child's difficulties. While some of these assessments include principles of neuropsychological assessment and intervention planning, not all do. In addition, even fewer of these screening and assessment strategies integrate tests of emotional and behavioral functioning and development.

This leaves teachers, parents, and clinicians at a disadvantage. While initial screening procedures may be helpful in identifying struggling students, they may be limited in their ability to be useful in developing interventions. Educators, therapists, parents, and school staff are often well-intentioned but they are also often at a disadvantage, lacking the time and resources to not only screen and assess their students but to develop interventions that directly correlate to a child's unique neuropsychological and emotional profile.

The intent of this manual is to provide a resource for clinicians, teachers, and specialists to make use of information garnered from comprehensive neuropsychological evaluations, which include psychological evaluations. Many people are involved in the process of evaluating students and then developing/implementing interventions. In this text, the term "specialist" refers to anyone involved in this process that is not a clinician or teacher. This includes but is not limited to: occupational therapists, speech therapists, outside consultants, reading and math remediation instructors, other school therapists and special education staff. The unfortunate and frequent gap between evaluation recommendations and implementation of interventions is largely due to the fact that specialists and teachers do not always have the time or means to both interpret and consistently apply these recommendations over the course of a school year. This manual will provide activities that are at the ready to address the various needs of students who present with learning disabilities and emotional or behavioral difficulties. In order to address the inherent overlap between academic, cognitive, social, and emotional development, tenets of attachment theory (Bowlby, 1988) and the ideas of Winnicott (1965) will be applied to the method of delivery and individualization of various interventions.

The importance of assessing emotional factors is increasingly recognized. Various studies have demonstrated that social-emotional competencies are important skills that support early school success and growth of academic competency in early grades (Denham et al., 2012; Jennings & DiPrete, 2010; Romano et al., 2010). The emotional state of an individual impacts their ability to regulate behaviors related to learning, classroom readiness, and deployment of attention (Bierman et al., 2008; McClelland et al., 2007). For example, children who have difficulties regulating negative emotions may not have the coping strategies to focus on learning activities, whereas those who can maintain a positive emotional state might be able to stay on task and remain engaged in academic activities (Graziano et al., 2007; Miller et al., 2006; Shields et al., 2001; Trentacosta & Izard, 2007). This is related to the child's emotional awareness and ability to identify their feelings and feelings of others.

This intrapersonal and interpersonal ability allows the child to interpret emotions in a classroom setting and comprehend the actions of others. Without these skills, the child may feel confused and overwhelmed. It has been demonstrated that this relationship between emotional/social awareness is connected to preschoolers' academic readiness (Garner & Waajid, 2008; Leerkes et al., 2008; Shields et al., 2001). These social-emotional skills are correlated to later school successes such as developing reading skills and overall academic achievement, as well as later social-emotional health (Denham et al., 2014). It can be argued that assessments of school-aged children should not only include their cognitive skills but also their social-emotional abilities, as assessed by psychological evaluations (Reinstein & Burau, 2014).

Over the last 15 years, the need for the integration of psychological and neuropsychological assessments has been argued by a number of authors (Semrud-Clickman et al., 1997; Smith, 2007; Tramontana & Hooper, 1997; Miller, 2010; Reinstein & Burau, 2014). Without an appreciation of the complex interplay between neurological, cognitive, behavioral, social, and emotional factors, treatment teams cannot develop interventions that address the whole child, creating a space in which the child feels safe and secure and can ultimately succeed (Reinstein & Burau, 2014). This reinforces the concept that utilizing neuropsychological assessments in a school setting cannot be viewed as a luxury but rather as essential to accurate diagnosis and treatment planning (Cleary & Scott, 2011). That said, many schools are at a disadvantage in the way in which children are evaluated, due to increasingly limited resources.

A variety of assessments are often used to determine a student's eligibility for special education services. Among the battery of tests, often neuropsychological evaluations provide important information/diagnoses for a student. However, it can be difficult to formally integrate information and recommendations into the legal documents that provide students with what they need. Recommendations for services such as individual remediation, special tutoring, the presence of an aide, or access to a resource room can be made in a neuropsychological evaluation and followed by schools, but how are the discrete cognitive and emotional functions reflected in legal documents?

In an attempt to narrow the gap between available resources, time, and implementation of interventions, this manual is intended to be a reference, providing teachers, clinicians, and parents with activities that can align with the results of integrated neuropsychological and psychological evaluations. In order to utilize this manual, it will be necessary to have a solid understanding of neuropsychological constructs, language, and evaluation results. The activities discussed throughout this manual are intended to be delivered through a relational perspective.

Before we continue to learn about Leila, it is important to understand the history and current process through which children are evaluated and the subsequent trends in intervention in a public school setting.

Response to Intervention

In 2004, the Individuals with Disabilities Education Improvement Act (IDEIA) became the nation's special education law. This law requires states to provide free appropriate public education (FAPE) in a least-restrictive environment (LRE) for all children regardless of the type of disability they may experience. This includes children with learning disabilities, as well as those with a severe, pervasive, and/or chronic emotional/affective condition that impacts their ability to perform everyday tasks (Sulkowski et al., 2011). Prior to the IDEIA, the law required the use of a "discrepancy model" for identifying struggling students (Hoover et al., 2008). This method often relied on a student's inability to perform at grade level despite the expectation they were capable of doing so. With the legal reform of 2004, educators and researchers began to develop new means for screening, assessing, and developing interventions for struggling students. This reform also established the requirement for the development of an Individualized Education Program (IEP) for individuals who qualify for special education services. This legal document outlines the type of educational program the student will have access to, and various accommodations, and determines clear annual goals with benchmarks. The intent of the document is to ensure that the student will have the best possible access to state curriculum or the federal guidelines, the Common Core State Standards (CCSS). Issues related to the development of IEPs and CCSS will be addressed in Chapter 9.

Response to Intervention (RTI) has become the most well-known systematic approach for attempting to provide FAPE for students with special needs. A 2011 survey was conducted by GlobalScholar in which, among nearly 1,400 school- and district-level workers, 68% indicated they have either partial or full districtwide implementation of the RTI model, particularly at the elementary grade level (Shah, 2011). Such studies display the heavy prevalence of this model within the public school system.

RTI was developed to provide a framework for providing all students with evidence-based instruction as well as ongoing measurements of their performance (Parisi et al., 2014). This framework has three intentions: (1) making instruction decisions in all classrooms; (2) determining eligibility for special education services; and (3) providing a system for identifying learning disabilities without relying on a discrepancy model (Hoover et al., 2008). To do so, entire student populations are screened/assessed three times a year, using assessments that are brief and easy to administer. If a student is identified as struggling, intervention can be made on a three-tier system that provides various levels of intervention. The student is then reassessed, as all the students are, after having access to the appropriate tiered level of support to determine the effectiveness of the intervention. If the intervention has proven ineffective, the student can then receive services from a more intensive tier (Parisi et al., 2014). For example, Tier 1 allows for changes and additional support within the general education classroom. Tier 2 allows for more intensive and individualized interventions, such as pull-out reading groups or tutoring, if the student continues to demonstrate significant difficulty. Tier 3 allows for students to have access to more highly specialized instruction and individualized interventions, such as a participation in a substantially separate classroom within a public school.

This systematic approach can be useful and moves away from the discrepancy model, but the extent of its efficacy is still being determined. For example, additional research is needed to document the usefulness of RTI in the later elementary, middle, and high school years (Otaiba et al., 2014). More so, while there is a preponderance of research regarding reading disabilities and RTI (especially at elementary grades), there are fewer studies related to disabilities of mathematics and emotional/behavioral difficulties. Under current laws and use of RTI, students with anxiety generally must fail to respond to evidence-based interventions before qualifying with an Emotional Disturbance allowing them access to higher-tiered intervention. At times, these students are assessed outside of the school setting to establish the presence of an anxiety disorder, but because the assessment does not directly indicate how the emotional difficulty affects the child's educational performance, there is no impact on the provision of services at school (Sulkowski et al., 2011). Furthermore, different schools utilize different assessment strategies and techniques. This can be a strength of RTI, avoiding a one-size-fits-all mentality, but how are assessments chosen and how is the data utilized? School psychologists and school neuropsychologists have indicated that the brief screening/assessment strategy may be too brief, unable to capture important nuances of a child's learning profile that could impact decisions regarding intervention strategies (Cleary & Scott, 2011). It is the lack of integration across grades, disabilities, service providers, and depth of assessment within and outside of school settings that create gaps that students can slip through, damaging their ability to access curriculum, develop a sense of self, and foster social relationships.

Furthermore, is RTI able to effectively guide intervention? While this model strives to assess the effectiveness of intervention, does it provide enough information to inform individualization of curriculum delivery? Or indicate the emotional needs of a child? Mascolo et al. (2014) propose a system springing from RTI that allows for the careful selection of intervention and treatment planning that includes a system for tailoring interventions to the unique strengths and vulnerabilities of a child. This system is based in the Cattell-Horn-Carroll (CHC) theory of intelligence. This approach carefully integrates various cognitive domains, but it does not integrate a child's emotional or behavioral profile into the process of tailoring interventions. As referenced above, Sulkowski et al. (2011) have described how RTI can be applied in school to address anxiety. However, this is not common practice. In fact, they note the disconnect between outside evaluations and implementation of interventions:

> It is important to note that psychologists who practice in clinical and community settings often produce psychological evaluations establishing the presence of anxiety disorders in youth. However, since this assessment may fail to establish how a disorder affects the child's educational performance or may lack important components that are mandated under IDEIA for special education eligibility (e.g., behavioral observations, teacher interviews), these evaluations may not impact the provision of services at school. For example, a school using RTI will require data establishing two criteria (e.g., functioning below peer-referenced norms and lack of adequate response to intervention) for eligibility. In cases where an outside evaluation supports the presence of a disorder that may impact a child's educational performance, pupil appraisal/IEP team members may decide to add the missing evaluation components to qualify a student to receive special education services under IDEIA. However, no mandate exists requiring these individuals to accept or follow diagnostic or treatment recommendations proposed by outside professionals, especially if there is an absence of corroborating data from different environments (e.g., home, school, community). (p. 942)

This situation exists for the many complex emotional conditions with which children are currently struggling. More often, emotional issues that impact behavior in school are addressed through behavioral interventions that are based on a Functional Behavioral Analysis (FBA). However, a number of studies question whether FBA utilization is appropriate for children with primary diagnoses of emotional difficulties (Sasso et al., 2001) and that its applicability is more appropriate for externalizing problems (aggression, property destruction) rather than internalizing problems (socially withdrawn behavior, obsessive behavior, symptoms of depression). Thus, according to Gable et al. (2014, p. 111), "there is more to learn about FBA in applied settings."

Given that the application of an FBA and subsequent utilization of traditional Applied Behavioral Analysis (ABA) techniques to address emotionally based difficulties continue to be a work in progress (Gable et al., 2014), there has been a movement in the behavioral field towards a Positive Behavioral Support system (Waguespack et al., 2006), including a three-tiered, School-Wide Positive Behavioral Support approach (Sugai & Horner, 2006). However, Waguespack et al. (2006) also acknowledge that these approaches continue to be a work in progress and that there is a need for further empirical studies, particularly in respect to the research-to-practice gap. Among other recommendations, they suggest that there needs to be an increased focus on prevention and tiered intervention, a shift away from the more traditional emphasis on consequent-based interventions and an increased emphasis on a team approach.

There are limitations to a behavioral approach that addresses a child's emotional difficulties which impede access to curriculum. It is time to consider an approach that is less focused on behavioral analysis and more focused on an understanding of behavior as a form of communication. This communication is concerned with underlying emotional and neurologically based difficulties, particularly maladaptive behaviors, which interfere with learning. We would contend that emotional distress drives maladaptive behaviors and this distress, within the school environment, is often a result of school-based environmental demands that impinge on a child's neurological or psychological vulnerabilities. To get at these vulnerabilities, one must peel back the behavioral and emotional layers within the context of a safe, secure, and nurturing relationship. It is essential that as teachers or support staff develop these relationships with their students, they be well-informed about underlying issues, specifically information gleaned from a comprehensive evaluation of neuropsychological and emotional functioning. Only then, with this level of understanding, can interventions be targeted and optimized to help students reach their full potential.

Although most commonly used within the current educational milieu, RTI and FBAs provide limited information and are not easily applied to the underlying emotional and neuropsychological difficulties that interfere with a child's learning. The following section describes a model that was developed as a framework in which neurological, emotional, social, and behavioral layers were addressed within the context of relationships. While, at times, there was data available that was based on a neuropsychological or psychological evaluation, the model that was employed allowed for an ongoing diagnostic process that took into account not only the behavioral domain, but the social, emotional, and neurological as well. This process was always rooted within the context of the relationships established with both the children and their families.

Here, we pick up the story of Leila. The results of a comprehensive neuropsychological evaluation present information on both her cognitive and emotional functioning, allowing for meaningful intervention to occur.

Cognitive testing with the WISC-V revealed that Leila's working memory was a relative weakness compared to other cognitive domains. The following table briefly outlines the results of the WISC-V:

	Score	*Percentile*
Verbal Comprehension	*133*	*99*
Visual Spatial	*135*	*99*
Fluid Reasoning	*131*	*98*
Working Memory	*97*	*42*
Processing Speed	*123*	*94*

These results suggest that while Leila is very bright, she struggles with holding information in her mind and manipulating it to meet the demands of an assignment or request. To a degree, this explained some of the cognitive rigidity observed in the classroom. Furthermore, while she had superior scores in visual spatial processing, as demonstrated by the Rey–Osterrieth Complex Figure Test (ROCF), vulnerabilities in Leila's executive functions, such as impulsivity and distractibility, impacted her performance. When graphomotor skills are involved, her performance is further impacted. This partially explained her difficulty with handwriting.

To better understand Leila's vulnerabilities around executive functions, she completed three subtests of the D-KEFS. Results indicated strengths in verbal fluency but significant difficulty with shifting cognitive set and monitoring her performance. She struggled with tasks that required inhibition and instead responded impulsively. The TOVA was used to further assess Leila's ability to deploy attentional skills and the results were consistent with individuals diagnosed with ADHD. Despite her weakness with working memory, all other memory tests, both visual and verbal, indicated results in the high average to very superior ranges, revealing memory as a great strength.

As part of the test battery, Leila's ability to perform academic skills was also assessed using the Woodcock Johnson III – Tests of Achievement. Results indicated that her Broad Reading Skills, Broad Math, Academic Fluency, and Academic Applications were all between the 69th and 78th percentile. However, her Broad Written Language skills were in the 23rd percentile. This indicates that while Leila is managing to apply her cognitive skills to learning in an academic environment, she struggles specifically with written output. Individual subtests revealed other strengths and vulnerabilities, but she specifically struggled with tasks that rely on certain types of fluency, spelling, and graphomotor output.

Leila's emotional well-being was assessed using the BASC-2, a Rorschach, and a series of projective assessments. Both parents and teachers indicated they were concerned about Leila's self-control, executive functions, modulation of negative feelings, hyperactivity, and aggression. Her teacher also noted concerns regarding depression. Leila herself indicated concerns about feeling hyperactive. It was also revealed that Leila demonstrated an average ability to read and articulate most affective facial expressions, but that she had difficulty integrating the angry affect of others into her perceptions. In a one-to-one setting, she could take the perspective of another, but in a larger group she could become emotionally overwhelmed and struggle to understand what other people were thinking and feeling. Leila had an awareness of some of her struggles, but did not know how to modulate the frustration level that could result from some of her vulnerabilities. Consequently, she could become defensive and angry and attempt to cover her vulnerabilities by appearing overconfident. This resulted in social difficulties, anxiety, and depression.

The results of the assessment were shared with Leila's parents, school, and, in a developmentally appropriate way, with Leila. The parents and school staff agreed that the information in the report described the child they had been observing for years. A better understanding of Leila's unique learning and social and emotional profile clarified the root of some of Leila's behaviors in the school setting. Now that there was a clear understanding, adjustments could be made in how academic material was presented, how teachers and staff responded to Leila in times of upset, and how to help Leila interact with people. Leila began individual therapy and the therapist worked closely with school staff to create an integrated approach. In therapy, Leila revealed that she "never learned the rules to life when other people just seem to know them." As a result, she was often confused and upset by the behaviors of others and didn't understand why she didn't know how to behave or why her reactions could be so extreme. At school, the staff was no longer concerned that Leila was becoming a bully or spoiled, but rather saw her as a child who required a compassionate approach to learning the "Rules of Life."

Peeling Back the Layers

The above case example describes a child who was dealing with a degree of complexity that required a careful analysis at multiple levels. The neuropsychological evaluation that was performed allowed a consideration not only of her behavior, but uncovered the emotional, social, and neurological factors that were contributing to Leila's presentation. We refer to this as *peeling back the layers.* This provides an alternative to a behavioral approach that often follows RTI and FBAs.

A child's behavior must be considered as a form of communication, one that requires a careful look at what lies underneath the child's attempt to convey some level of distress. While an FBA may be successful at identifying antecedent conditions and consequences, the driving forces behind behavior that is analyzed at this level are almost always described as either avoidance of a task or an attempt to gain attention. Although this level of understanding is sufficient to develop a detailed chart or graph, it remains on the surface and does not address underlying factors; factors that almost always include significant neurological or emotional issues or some combination of both. Furthermore, an RTI approach would merely delay a deeper understanding of why Leila was behaving as she was. Clearly, many interventions had been attempted over the years, but none was dispelling the growing feeling and perception on the part of the school that she was "mean, spoiled, and selfish" and would need a different school placement. A comprehensive neuropsychological evaluation, including a careful analysis of her emotional functioning, allowed the creation of a different narrative. This new narrative dispelled the negative perceptions of those around Leila and allowed for a more compassionate and inclusive approach to supporting her in school.

"Peeling back the layers" describes a process of questioning, examining, and weighing findings that have been evaluated at the levels of behavioral, social, emotional, and neurological functioning. Once information has been gathered from each of these layers through a neuropsychological assessment, the findings are then integrated to create a description of the *whole child* and formulate recommendations for them (Reinstein & Burau, 2014). This approach assumes that a child's behavior is a form of communication that evolves because the child does not possess the skills to communicate important information more directly. This important information is ultimately related to an emotional response to perceived demands placed on him/her. These demands are placed on a child by both his/her internal and external environments. In respect to the former, internal demands may be placed by a child herself who, for example, expects her performance to be perfect or is aware that she is not adequately managing the social scene. In the case of the latter, these could include academic demands within the school or within the context of school work at home. They could also include classroom demands to sit still at a desk, keep up with the social conversation of peers, engage in age-appropriate play, accurately perceive social cues, and so forth. Additional external demands may be a corollary to a home environment that is, itself, disruptive.

When a child experiences himself or herself as not meeting one or more of these demands, they can become anxious, sad, angry, or all of the above and tend to externalize or internalize these emotions. These feelings can then drive behaviors that cover a spectrum of acting out angrily or disruptively, as did Leila, or withdrawing and becoming increasingly socially isolated. Without an understanding of the source of a child's emotional response, one cannot effectively address the behavior in a meaningful and long-lasting way.

Getting below the behavioral layer to the emotional and social layers is but the first step. One must continue to question whether or not there is another layer that is neurologically based. This is a question that is best addressed through a careful assessment of neurological functioning, which might initially include results from a neuropsychological evaluation that looks at cognition, executive functions, memory abilities, and visual motor skills, among others. Vulnerabilities in one or more of these areas can be experienced by a child as a deficit that impairs their functioning and, without a more specific understanding of their relative strengths and vulnerabilities, creates the impression that they are damaged in some manner. Many children, even those who have very significant areas of strength, can begin to question their abilities in a more global fashion once they begin to bump up against a vulnerability that can make them feel different and less able. Such a neurologically based struggle can create an emotional reaction that impacts the child socially and behaviorally, creating multiple layers of defense as a means to protect themselves. Thus the process of reversing this order, by peeling back the layers, attempts to identify the root cause of behavior that is a communication about that underlying root issue. Managing behavior or experimenting with interventions without a clear understanding of the root and resultant defenses can be ineffective or, worse yet, exacerbate the situation by contributing to the frustration and sense of failure, not only for the child, but for the service provider as well. As in the case of Leila, it can lead to the impulse to give up.

Once the layers are peeled back and there is some additional data about underlying causes, what does one do with this information? In the next section, we will discuss how one can integrate an understanding of the difficulties a child is facing within the context of a relational approach to remediation.

Developing a Therapeutic Relationship

When we talk about a therapeutic relationship, we are doing so primarily as it relates to the teachings of Donald W. Winnicott and John Bowlby and how they have been integrated into the philosophy we have developed at the Community Therapeutic Day School, or CTDS (Reinstein, 2006).

Donald Winnicott was a psychiatrist in London, England, who worked with children beginning in the 1930s until his death in 1971. As part of the British psychoanalytic movement, he put into practice the approach of the object relations school of psychoanalytic thought. This approach was based on the belief that a child's development proceeded within the context of a relationship, specifically the relationship of the developing child to an object (a perhaps unfortunate term to describe a person other than the child). Winnicott described three main principles defining the manner in which this development took place. The first was the belief in the natural unfolding of the developmental process. This meant that each child possessed the inherent capacity to develop towards physical and emotional maturity as long as the environment supported her growth. The second principle he described as the *good enough* mother (or primary caretaker). This was an attempt to acknowledge that there was no *ideal* mother, but rather, that a child could develop well within a relationship that was a good enough match between child and mother, one that took into account a particular child's needs and the ability of the caretaker to sufficiently meet those needs. The third principle was the concept of the *holding environment*. As delineated by Winnicott, the holding environment described the quality of the developing caretaker–child relationship and the space in which it unfolded. It included the ability of the caretaker to recognize the child's specific physical, psychological, and emotional needs and to provide a safe and consistent environment that was capable of adjusting to the moment-to-moment needs of the child. Thus, the holding environment was one in which the child felt seen, acknowledged, and safely held within a relationship that facilitated their growth (Reinstein, 2006).

John Bowlby, a psychologist, was a contemporary of Winnicott in London and also a part of the British Psychoanalytic Society within the object relations movement. He too focused on the relationship between the mother and child over the course of the child's development. Bowlby was heavily influenced by the field of ethology and derived the idea that, in humans, there was an instinctual drive for a child to attach to a primary caretaker as a means towards survival. As he noted,

> Attachment behaviour is any form of behaviour that results in a person attaining or maintaining proximity to some other clearly identified individual who is conceived as better able to cope with the world. It is most obvious whenever the person is frightened, fatigued or sick and is assuaged by comforting and caregiving.
>
> (Bowlby, 1988, p. 27)

Bowlby went further on to explain that "There is abundant evidence that almost every child habitually prefers one person, usually his mother-figure, to whom to go when distressed but that, in her absence, he will make do with someone else, preferably someone whom he knows well" (ibid., p. 28).

Attachment behaviors typically begin in infancy and communicate to the primary caregiver that the child desires their close proximity. Behaviors such as crying and rooting or sucking might indicate distress or hunger. Smiling and babbling indicate the desire for social interaction with the primary caregiver (Bowlby, 1982). In these examples, the attuned caregiver will understand the need of the child and attempt to meet it to the best of their ability. The crying child is bounced to provide proprioceptive input, the diaper is changed, or they are fed. There are clear needs with clear responses that result in a soothing effect. As the child grows, attachment behaviors change and become more sophisticated and the responses of the caregiver in turn change to meet the changing needs of the child.

For most children, the classroom constitutes an environment in which the focus is academic and any minor behavioral, social, and/or emotional issues take a back seat. For such a child, their relationship with a teacher, while important, is not crucial. For a child with significant learning, behavioral, social, and/or emotional difficulties, however, the level of distress that they experience within the classroom can be overwhelming. Consequently, school is experienced as neither safe nor consistent and a child with these significant issues will not feel seen, acknowledged, or accommodated, despite good efforts by the teacher or school staff. As such, the classroom does not provide a holding environment for the child. Furthermore, the child's emotional and behavioral response to distress, without a deeper understanding of the root cause on the part of teachers and specialists, can disrupt the development of a relationship with the teacher. This disruption can result in a relationship that is no longer ***good enough*** for the child to access learning in a way that her cognitive development unfolds naturally. This child, because of the level of distress, desperately needs an attachment figure, someone who can comfort and reassure them that they are seen, their difficulties are acknowledged, and there will be steps taken to ensure that accommodations will be made so that they can resume on the path to learning and growth.

With the results of a comprehensive neuropsychological evaluation that integrates emotional/social functioning, inexplicable behaviors can become clearer. The process of peeling back the layers can reveal the root cause of the behaviors, which could now be viewed as ***attachment behaviors***, or a means for communicating a need that has been unmet. For children with a variety of disabilities, their methods of communication can be confusing and the method for meeting their need may be unusual or difficult to identify. The results of a comprehensive neuropsychological evaluation can be used to identify clues that explain the child's behavior and decode the attachment behaviors the child displays, providing insight into the type of intervention required for the child to feel safe, experience a consistent relationship within the classroom, and develop a holding environment.

Examples of attachment behaviors during infancy were described above (crying, rooting, smiling), but what do these behaviors look like in older children and how do they relate to neuropsychological functioning? As educators, clinicians, and parents, the more familiar we become with the various neuropsychological functional domains (see Box 1.1) the easier it is to identify how they impact functionality in a variety of settings. In the following chapters, each functional domain will be discussed and tables explaining how each domain can be observed or expressed through behaviors and social interactions will be presented. This knowledge can then inform adults as to what interventions to supply, how to relate to the student, and how to develop a holding environment tailored to the needs of the individual within a group. This approach is beneficial in that, once attachment behaviors based in neuropsychological findings are identified, interventions from various theoretical and educational origins can be applied and interventions are not restricted to one approach. This can include behavioral approaches, various educational paradigms, gestalt theory, person-centered theory, expressive therapies, and so on.

Box 1.1 Functional Domains

Cognitive Skills

Executive Functions

Memory

Visual Motor Skills

Academic Skills

Emotional/Behavioral

Inclusion Possibilities

This relational approach to education is not limited to the treatment of an individual, but can be applied to the classroom or to entire programs. Between 1995 and 2009, the CTDS Inclusion program successfully supported over 40 public school children from kindergarten through high school. The program was designed to address each child's unique academic, behavioral, social, and emotional needs. This was a model designed and implemented previously in another Boston-area town and, for both towns, was described in detail in a previous publication (Reinstein, 2006). The unique accommodations provided for each child were implemented within very specific frameworks that were dictated by the age and severity of need for each. For example, at the elementary level, approximately 70% of the children were included in mainstream classrooms with support. However, we were also able to accommodate children with more severe needs in substantially separate therapeutic classrooms. Once at the middle and high school levels, these children employed a Therapeutic Resource Room model and were mainstreamed for academic classes. The strategies and techniques utilized provided a holding environment (Winnicott, 1965) that was primarily relationship-based but also drew on an eclectic mix of interventions.

The prime directive for each teacher or support staff was to honor and develop a relationship with the child and his or her parents. A team approach was used to integrate all aspects of the treatment plan, engaging the parents as well as any outside service providers. A case manager was designated as the one responsible for coordinating treatment with the child and family. Each child was seen in weekly psychotherapy and parents met or spoke with the case manager on a weekly basis. A communication notebook went back and forth between home and school daily and included information about the child's day/evening with a particular emphasis on the emotional and behavioral issues with which he or she was struggling. Furthermore, communication between team members was frequent to ensure that all involved were consistent in their approach. For example, all of the team members were supervised weekly by the clinical psychologist to evaluate and update ongoing interventions and to support the members of each teaching unit. These meetings were also used to assess working diagnoses and make recommendations about any additional assessments that would inform changes on any of the various layers being considered. Thus, a holding environment was constructed to support the team and integrate treatment across school and home. In this way, the children and their families felt held and engaged in the ongoing support and treatment.

This highly integrated and coordinated approach sent a message to the child that they would be seen and provided with an environment in which their complex needs could be met, rather than focusing on managing behavior at a superficial level. While many of the children were on the higher-functioning end of the autism spectrum, the program also included children with complex psychiatric diagnoses such as bipolar disorder, anxiety disorder, attachment disorder, obsessive compulsive disorder, intermittent explosive disorder, schizophrenia, depression, ADHD, or some combination of those. Using this approach, the program was able to maintain these children within the public school system and provide them with a successful school experience. For example, a cohort of children was followed from as early as kindergarten through high school and, at one point, all eight of the children at the high school level made the honor roll. While this level of success was certainly not a guarantee for all of the children in the program, it does speak to the way in which this approach enabled each child to demonstrate their potential.

A Guide to Integrating Neuropsychological, Psychological Result and Relational Education

Box 1.2

Introduction
Observing Functional Domain
Observation and Development of Functional Domain
Developing Accommodations and Interventions General Academic Accommodations and Strategies
Addressing Functional Domain
Intro to the interventions and activities with general recommendations
Functional Domain General Interventions and Activities
Social/Emotional
Academic
Environmental Considerations
Other Services (if applicable)
Chapter Appendix

This manual is intended to act as a guide for implementing assessment results using a relational approach. In Chapters 2 through 6, more specific approaches and strategies are delineated to address specific learning, behavioral, social, and emotional difficulties. Each of these chapters follows a similar organizational structure (see Box 1.2). A short introduction describing the specific functional domain is followed by a section describing how that particular domain might be observed in the child's behavior at school or in the home. Then, developmental tables describe how that domain might manifest over the child's preschool and school years. Assessment tools used to measure each functional domain are included in the charts. Possible interventions or accommodations appropriate for use in the classroom, on IEPs, or on 504 plans are then presented. Next is a section that focuses on specific interventions for that domain which include considerations of social/emotional, academic, and environmental factors. Lastly, each of these five chapters includes an appendix that provides specific activities which support growth in the given domain. Thus, chapters 2–7 follow the general outline in Box 1.2. The final two chapters focus on the development of an IEP and working with families.

–2–

Cognitive Interventions

Introduction

In this chapter, we will consider how findings from a neuropsychological evaluation can be implemented to address cognitive vulnerabilities. We will also consider what kind of questions one could pose and how observations at school and in the home can be used to begin to identify areas of vulnerability within the cognitive domain. As noted previously (Reinstein & Burau, 2014), attempting to delineate cognition as a separate functional domain is an artificial construct, as cognition is inextricably intertwined with all other domains and is only one dimension of the "whole child." Consequently, this discussion will invariably touch on the other domains discussed in more detail in subsequent chapters.

When we talk about cognition within this context, we are considering both verbal and non-verbal intellectual functioning. To a degree, this is largely framed by the fact that both neuropsychological and academic assessments somewhat narrowly identify these domains as relevant to the learning process. Thus, for our purposes, cognition or intelligence is defined as "the ability to adjust or adapt to the environment, the ability to learn, or the ability to perform abstract thinking (e.g., to use symbols and concepts)" (Sattler, 2008, p. 224). Within the construct of neuropsychological testing and academics, the verbal and non-verbal domains are assessed by tests of intelligence, such as the Wechsler Intelligence Scale for Children, Fifth Edition (WISC-V), the Stanford-Binet Intelligence

Scale, Fifth Edition (SB-5), the Kaufman Assessment Battery for Children, Second Edition (KABC-II), or the Woodcock-Johnson, Fourth Edition, Cognitive (WJ-IV-COG). For the sake of brevity, we will consider both verbal and non-verbal intelligence as measured by the WISC-V. For a more in-depth discussion of these assessment batteries, the reader is directed to Reinstein and Burau (2014).

The Verbal Comprehension Index on the WISC-V is a composite of scores from two subtests. These tests largely relate to the functioning of the left hemisphere of the brain and, as such, reflect the processing of both receptive and expressive language skills. The Vocabulary subtest is a measure of word knowledge, assessing a child's ability to define words of increasing difficulty. It evaluates verbal comprehension, language development, and the ability to understand abstract language concepts. The Similarities subtest measures verbal concept formation and requires that the child describe how two conceptually related words are alike as they progress from more concrete and experientially based ideas to increasingly abstract concepts. Among other things, it measures a child's verbal comprehension, ability to understand relationships, conceptual thinking, use of logic, and abstraction (Wechsler, 2014).

Visual Spatial Organization, or right-hemisphere non-verbal skills, is measured by the Block Design and Visual Puzzles subtests of the WISC-V. These skills allow one to negotiate the non-verbal visual spatial world or the world that is not processed in a linear, language-based manner. The Block Design subtest is a timed test that requires the child to recreate a two-dimensional design using two-color blocks. It measures the ability to analyze and synthesize abstract visual information, non-verbal concept formation and reasoning, visual perception and organization as well as visual-motor coordination. The Visual Puzzles subtest, administered within time limits, requires that the child view a two-dimensional puzzle and select three response options out of six that, when combined, reconstruct the puzzle. It measures mental constructive abilities that are not dependent on a motor response, visual and spatial reasoning, the understanding of part-to-whole relationships, and the analysis and synthesis of abstract visual stimuli (Wechsler, 2014).

Fluid Reasoning is measured by two subtests of the WISC-V which assess a child's ability to perceive underlying conceptual relationships between visual objects by using logic to identify and apply rules. In Matrix Reasoning, an untimed test, the child observes an incomplete visual grid or sequence and selects a response from five options that completes the design. The child uses visual-spatial abilities to discern the underlying conceptual rule, which requires fluid intelligence. The Figure Weights subtest is completed within time limits and calls for the child to view a series of scales with missing weights and select a response from five options that keeps the scale balanced. It is a measure of quantitative fluid reasoning and emphasizes inductive or deductive logical thought (Wechsler, 2014).

Observing Cognitive Functions

Whether it's in a classroom setting, the therapist's office or in a car on the ride home from an activity, we can observe a child and note their strengths and vulnerabilities in both the verbal and non-verbal cognitive realms. In order to recognize cognitive functioning in any environment, we can train ourselves to ask certain questions as we observe the child. The following list is a good starting point for questions to consider in the various cognitive domains.

Verbal Comprehension

What is their rate of speech?

Does their vocabulary seem age-appropriate? Advanced? Behind?

Do they have difficulty drawing inferences?

Do they enjoy having conversations or do they choose to participate in other activities?

Are they aware of interrupting others or oneself?

Do they often veer off topic or have "random" responses to questions?

Are they tangential?

Do they struggle with oral expression, including word retrieval and organization of thoughts?

Are they able to stop talking when asked?

Do they take turns in conversations or tend to monologue?

Do they have a tendency to stay on one topic even when others have changed topics?

Do they get easily confused when other people are speaking?

Do they understand metaphors and similes?

Do they have a tendency to literally interpret language? Can they use precise language to effectively communicate ideas?

Do they struggle to determine operations in mathematical word problems?

Do they struggle with automatizing the relationship between numbers and words?

Do they struggle with fluency or word retrieval while reading?

Do they have difficulty including a variety of words or vocabulary while writing? Are their sentences redundant?

Visual Spatial

Do they enjoy puzzles? Tangrams?

Do they like to construct things using their hands such as towers, two-dimensional images or collages?

When playing games like Where's Waldo?, how quickly do they find objects? Do they get frustrated easily? Do they enjoy these sorts of activities?

Do they have difficulty staying within margins or drawing in a specified space?

How quickly do they learn to read maps or identify locations on maps?

When interacting socially, do they appear confused by the expressions, gestures, and non-verbal communication of other people?

Do they have difficulty perceiving relationships between patterns?

Fluid Reasoning

How does the child respond to novel situations? Do they become distracted, shut down, or rigid?

Do they have difficulty understanding relationships between new concepts?

When presented with new academic material, how much scaffolding is required to help them integrate it into an existing body of information?

Do they have a limited ability to problem-solve in everyday situations?

Do they have problems understanding and evaluating opinions of others?

Do they struggle with math problems that integrate a variety of concepts that might include number sense, estimation, fractions, integers, etc.?

Do they have difficulty representing numbers or problems in a variety of ways?

Do they have poor inferential or predictive skills while reading?

Do they grasp the main idea of a reading selection?

Can they understand that the audience or reader may have a different point of view and purpose than their own?

Can they make sense of rules to games that require reasoning based on verbal information, such as I Spy or 20 Questions?

Can they make sense of visual elimination games such as Guess Who?, Battleship, and Mastermind?

Can they find the rules to a pattern?

When given a problem to solve, do they understand the rules of the problem and the limitation of possible responses?

Observation and Development of Cognitive Functions

The following charts outline how verbal, visual spatial, and fluid reasoning may appear as observable behaviors. Bear in mind that cognitive skills have a developmental trajectory and that, when making observations, age, experience, and exposure should be considered. To that point, the behaviors listed in the charts start with the behaviors of a two-year-old child and continue through 18 years. In addition to observable behaviors, the charts include assessment tools that can be used at various developmental points to evaluate the designated skills.

Verbal Functioning

The development of verbal functioning relies on more than just the use of words. It also includes the pragmatics and semantic elements of language as well as syntax and phonology. For example, a five-year-old child might be able to recite the Magna Carta, but they have no ability to comprehend the meaning. This child has good phonology and clearly a strong verbal memory, but the ability to comprehend the complex vocabulary and concepts within the Magna Carta has not developed.

TABLE 2.1 Verbal Functioning Development

Age	*Expressive*	*Receptive*	*Assessments*
2–2:6 years	• Uses 3-word sentences • Refers to self as "me" • Use of simple questions (what, who, where) • Uses "and" • Narratives mostly labels and descriptions • **450+ words**	• Responds to location phrases (in, on) • Understands questions about objects (what), people (who), events (where is *x* going)	• Bayley Scales of Infant and Toddler Development, Third Edition (Bayley-III) • SB-5
2:6–3 years	• Answers questions with "yes" and "no" • Uses 3- to 4-word sentences • Asks "wh" questions, "why" questions • Begins singular/plural noun-verb agreement • Relates simple imaginative narratives • Uses basic spatial terms • Ability to produce rhyme • **900+ words**	• Understands "why" questions • Understands spatial terms (in, on, under) • Understands concepts of "one" and "all" • Interest in "why" and "how" explanations • Understands "now," "soon," and "later" • Follows 2-step commands	• Bayley-III • SB-5 • Wechsler Preschool and Primary Scale of Intelligence, Fourth Edition (WPPSI-IV) • WJ-IV
3 4 years	• Uses pronouns (we, she, they) • Expresses ideas and feelings • Begins using analogies • Describes use of objects • Begins complex sentences (4–5 words) • Can tell a story • **1500+ words**	• Enjoys poems • Recognizes language absurdities • Understands basic color, size, and shape words	• Bayley-III (up to 42 months) • SB-5 • WPPSI-IV • WJ-IV • KABC-II
4–5 years	• Uses "when" and "how" questions • Asks "wh" do and "wh" did questions • Longer and more complex sentences • Uses conjunctions (and, because) • Uses comparative adjectives (big – bigger) • Ends conversations appropriately • **2,500 words**	• Follows 3-step commands • Identifies more colors and shapes • Understands "in the morning," "next," and "noontime" • Knowledge of letter names and sounds • Knowledge of numbers and counting emerges	• SB-5 • WPPSI-IV • WJ-IV • KABC-II

(continued)

TABLE 2.1 *(continued)*

Age	*Expressive*	*Receptive*	*Assessments*
5–6 years	• Uses complex and compound sentences with 8+ words • Stories have central focus, high point, and resolution • **5,000 words**	• Understands time sequences (what happened first, second, etc.) • Understands "same" and "different" • Understands common opposites	• SB-5 • WPPSI-IV • WJ-IV • KABC-II
6–9 years	• Stories with internal goals, motivations, and reactions of characters • Language used for social status • Increase in figurative language • Multiple meanings of words • Phonological knowledge for spelling		• WPPSI-IV (up to 7:7 years) • SB-5 • WJ-IV • KABC-II • WISC-V
9–12 years	• Vocabulary in text more abstract • New information from written text • Explains relationship between multiple meanings of words • Metacognitive skills emerge	• Understands jokes and riddles based on lexical ambiguity • Understands common idioms	• SB-5 • WJ-IV • KABC-II • WISC-V
12–14 years	• Abstract dictionary definitions for words • Explains meanings of proverbs • Syntax in writing more complex than in speech	• Understands jokes and riddles based on deep structure ambiguity	• SB-5 • WJ-IV • KABC-II • WISC-V
15–18 years	• Average vocabulary size of high school graduate (**10,000 words**) • Language used to maintain social bonds • Written language more complex than spoken • Adult range of syntactic constructions reached		• WISC-IV (up to 16:11 years) • SB-5 • WJ-IV • KABC-II

Sources: Brandon et al. (2006), LD Online (1999), First Years (2011).

Perceptual Reasoning

Perceptual reasoning skills have been studied from various perspectives (philosophy, psychology, neuroscience, etc.) for many years. Despite the wealth of research, a succinct developmental chart has not been developed. In more recent years, this task has been taken on by many theorists and scientists. The result is a nascent perspective on perceptual reasoning development. The study of perceptual reasoning development is further complicated by the overlap of nature and nurture. Multiple studies have demonstrated that human perceptual development is based in biological sensory systems and that the assigned meaning of the sensory input is rooted in culture, exposure, and experience. Further complicating the study of perceptual reasoning skills is the overlap with studies of neural, motor, cognitive, language, emotional, and social development (Bornstein, Arterberry, & Mash, 2011). Table 2.2 should be regarded as a guide for various aspects of perceptual reasoning skills as they are assessed in neuropsychological evaluations and which *may* be present in the natural environment. When viewing this table, bear in mind the previously identified complicating factors that may impact the development of these skills.

Fluid Reasoning

The study of the developmental course of fluid or abstract reasoning has its roots in observations made by the developmental psychologist Jean Piaget (1896–1980). He delineated four stages of cognitive development. In the sensorimotor stage (birth to 2 years), a child learns to interact with the physical world. In the pre-operational stage (2 to 7 years), the child learns to represent states mentally. In the concrete-operational stage (7 to 11 years), the child learns to manipulate mental representations internally. And in the last stage, formal operational (11 years onward), a child can reason with abstract possibilities, reason from hypotheses to deductions, and reason with propositions. Thus, according to Piaget, true abstract reasoning occurs in the last stage, formal operational, a development that takes place beginning at about 11 years of age.

Fluid reasoning has also been defined psychometrically and, for our purposes, we will consider how the development of abstract reasoning relates to the interface of observed behavior and assessment. Cattell (1971) identified fluid intelligence (Gf) as one of two factors, the other being crystallized intelligence (Gc), that together make up overall intelligence. Fluid intelligence was defined as the ability to reason in novel ways and entailed the ability to derive relations through inductive reasoning and reason abstractly. Consistent with Piagetian theory, Cattell, and Horn (1988), contended that fluid reasoning skills peak between the ages of 15 and 20. However, they also reported that aspects of fluid reasoning begin to emerge in the first two to three years of life. To a large extent, however, the ability to demonstrate fluid reasoning skills also depends on the emergence of working memory capacity, inhibitory control, and the ability to shift attention toward salient details and filter out non-relevant details (Krawczyk et al., 2010).

The chart below traces the development of fluid reasoning and is based on psychometric principles. It begins at 2 years as tests that measure fluid reasoning, for example, are included on the SB-5 at that age.

TABLE 2.2 Perceptual Reasoning Development

Age	*Visual Acuity and Development*	*Auditory Discrimination*	*Visual Spatial Organization*	*Test/Subtests*
2–3 years	20/20		Children begin building with blocks both horizontally and vertically, creating solid structures that have walls or floors	• Bayley-III • Differential Ability Scales, Second Edition (DAS-II) • WPPSI-IV • SB-5 • KABC-II • WJ-IV
3–4 years			Perception of color categories increases Begin building blocks in 3 dimensions, often creating piles of blocks with no interior Between the ages of 3 and 6, visual information becomes increasingly unnecessary for balance control and other perception-action coupled movements	• Bayley-III • DAS-II • WPPSI-IV • SB-5 • KABC-II • WJ-IV
4–5 years			Between the ages of 4 and 11, while perceiving that they are copying an actual object rather than a collection of lines, they attempt to copy the object and not the depicted lines Difficulty copying acute and obtuse angles	• DAS-II • WPPSI-IV • SB-5 • KABC-II • WJ-IV
5–7 years			Ability to draw closed shapes is different depending on the shape, struggling more with diamonds than squares More accurately reproduce symmetrical dotted patterns then asymmetrical ones	• DAS-II • WPPSI-IV (up to 7:7 years) • SB-5 • KABC-II • WJ-IV • WISC-V

7–9 years		Rapid improvement in depth perception and figure-ground perception, maturing by age 12	• DAS-II • WPPSI-IV (up to 7:7 years) • SB-5 • KABC-II • WJ-IV • WISC-V
9–11 years		Reproduce asymmetrical dotted patterns more accurately	• DAS-II • SB-5 • KABC-II • WJ-IV • WISC-V
11–13 years	Sensory abilities typically mature by puberty, but comprehensive perceptual functioning does not		
13–17 years		The onset of puberty correlates with a slight decrease in encoding unfamiliar faces. Adult level of facial encoding typically occurs around age 16	• DAS-II • SB-5 • KABC-II • WJ-IV • WISC-V
17 to Adult	Adults who speak tone languages (such as Mandarin Chinese) process pitch with greater accuracy than those who do not	Adults rely less on oscillating visual information to maintain balance and rely on other sensory systems	• Wechsler Adult Intelligence Scale Fourth Edition (WAIS-IV) • SB-5 • WJ-IV

Sources: Guanella (1934); Raskin et al. (1983); Lee (1989); Gallahue & Ozmun (2002); Pitchford & Mullen (2003); Smith (2003); Carey et al. (1980); Deutsch et al. (2004).

TABLE 2.3 Fluid Reasoning Development

Age	*Fluid Reasoning Behavior*	*Assessments*
2–4 years	• Symbolic representation • Simple pretend play to symbolic pretend play • Object constancy • Objects represented as pictures	• SB-5 (Fluid Reasoning – Verbal and Non-verbal) • DAS (Picture Similarities, Matrices)
4–5 years	• Theory of mind • Time concept • Generalizes rules	• SB-5 (same) • DAS (same) • WPPSI-IV (Matrix Reasoning, Picture Concepts) • WJ-IV-COG (Number Series, Concept Formation)
5–7 years	• Representational activity increases • Ability to represent objects in pictures increases • Pretend play (symbolic representation) increases in complexity	• SB-5 (same) • WPPSI-IV (same – up to 7 years) • WISC-V (Matrix Reasoning, Figure Weights; 6–16 years) • WJ-IV-COG (same)
7–11 years	• Thinking more flexible, logical and organized • Operational thinking reversible, more organized, and inter-connected • Logico-arithmetical operations (class inclusion, conservation, perspective-taking) • Spatial operations (distance, time, velocity, space) • Cannot do abstract operations	• SB-5 (same) • DAS (same) • WISC-V (same) • WJ-IV-COG (same)
11–17 years	• Ability to operate on operations • Reason with abstract possibilities • Form hypotheses and deduce using logic and test theories • Reason about logical relationships between propositions	• SB-5 (same) • DAS (same) • WISC-V (same) • WJ-IV-COG (same)

Source: Birney & Sternberg (2011).

Developing Accommodations and Interventions

Once a child's strengths and vulnerabilities in the cognitive realm have been identified through observation and assessment, accommodations can be put in place and interventions can be made to help support their strengths, circumvent challenges, promote a positive sense of self, and develop coping mechanisms. The following sections indicate specific interventions that can be made to address an individual's vulnerabilities and strengths. It is important to individualize the accommodations or interventions to the specific needs, characteristics, interests, and abilities of the individual or group. Also, bear in mind the importance of addressing both academic and social/emotional components of functioning. To that end, both academic and social/emotional interventions and accommodations will be presented. Some interventions and accommodations are appropriate at any age or grade level, as long as the delivery method and content is appropriate to their skill level. For example, a 10-year-old student who has strong verbal comprehension skills but weak phonological processing ability must develop phonological processing skills. It is important, however, to refrain from using books for younger children, as doing so will likely negatively impact their self-esteem. The initial list of accommodations is general and can be applied at most grade levels.

General Academic Accommodations and Strategies

The following list of accommodations and strategies can be implemented in the classroom. Some of these accommodations can be included in an IEP or 504 plan.

- Use both verbal and visual cues and schedules.
- Break tasks into subtasks with clear deadlines.
- Provide step-by-step directions.
- Provide lecture notes or recorded lectures.
- Provide extra time for tests and exams.
- Allow use of calculator.
- Avoid the use of figurative language when giving directions.
- Use social stories with simplified language and visual aids/images.
- Allow for interactive learning opportunities that engage multiple senses.

Verbal Comprehension General Accommodations

- Provide a glossary of important terms.
- Establish preferential setting near teacher.
- Provide visual cues and reminders.
  Give directions in written and verbal format.
- Use succinct and clear language, avoiding figurative language.
- Provide copy of written notes when presenting orally.

Verbal Comprehension Mathematics Accommodations

- Provide a number line on the child's desk.
- Provide step-by-step examples on the child's desk.
- Provide verbalization of each math step.
- Provide model at the top of worksheets.
- Use choral responding to questions.
- Develop verbal narrative of math steps.
- Reword math vocabulary in simpler terms.
- Modify word problems using simplified language.

- Reduce volume of writing and copying.
- Use cloze procedure on worksheets.
- Allow oral response.
- Provide math vocabulary reference sheet for tests and exams.

Verbal Comprehension Reading Accommodations

- Preview new words and pair with visual cues.
- Simplify complex text by rewording.
- Allow additional time to read.
- Highlight key words and concepts.
- Allow access to online books, electronic books, text reader (Reading Pen, Scan and Read) or electronic dictionary.
- Provide graphic organizers to highlight main ideas and key concepts.
- Provide alternative-format print materials.

Verbal Comprehension Writing Accommodations

- Allow access to word processor, digital notepad or voice recognition software.
- Use templates, graphic organizers and outlines.
- Reduce volume of note taking.
- Provide scribe for tests and exams.

Perpetual Reasoning General Accommodations

- If perceptual reasoning is a strength, use visual cues such as color coding and pictures in the environment and in academic work.
- If perceptual reasoning is a vulnerability, simplify the environment to be free of clutter. Reduce visual complexity on worksheets and other academic work.
- Provide step-by-step directions that are presented visually and verbally.
- Teach students to break large tasks into smaller steps.
- When copying information from a whiteboard, chalkboard, or Smart Board, provide a template for the student to fill in (cloze procedure).
- For left-handed students, provide worksheets with word banks in the right margin.
- Provide scribe when necessary.
- Use multiple choice and cloze procedure during test-taking. Avoid open-ended questions.

Perpetual Reasoning Mathematics Accommodations

- Reduce number of items on a page or worksheet.
- Provide lined paper or graph paper.
- Allow use of manipulative and concrete objects.
- Allow access to a number line.

Perpetual Reasoning Reading Accommodations

- Reduce number of items on a page or worksheet.

Perpetual Reasoning Writing Accommodations

- Allow access to word processing system.
- Provide extended time on writing assignments and exams.

Fluid Reasoning General Accommodations

- Explicitly teach multiple approaches to solving problems.
- Teach concrete concepts before abstract.
- Define relationships and connections between ideas in a concrete manner.
- Provide analogies and stories the individual can relate to or has experienced.
- Provide opportunities to sort, classify and categorize.
- Use a "think out loud" method of reasoning for problem-solving tasks to demonstrate the thought process.
- Use graphic organizers to assist in unifying information visually and verbally.
- Use cooperative groups and reciprocal teaching.
- Monitor student at a high rate to ensure and assess understanding of directions and concepts.
- Monitor functioning through a task and particularly when there are changes in demands.

Fluid Reasoning Mathematics Accommodations

- Teach math mnemonic strategies that specifically identify the steps for problem-solving.
- Teach patterns and relationships such as skip-counting or patterns in a 100 chart to help learn multiplication and other math facts and relationships.
- Attach a number line to the desk to help with number sense and pattern recognition.
- Provide manipulatives in order to help make information concrete and less abstract.
- Demonstrate explanation of problem-solving strategies, then ask the student to explain their strategies to the teacher or a peer.
- Allow use of calculator.

Fluid Reasoning Reading Accommodations

- Use graphic organizers to help summarize information.
- Model self-monitoring skills while reading, demonstrating how to ask oneself if material/words have been understood.
- Teach how to identify main ideas.

Fluid Reasoning Writing Accommodations

- Use graphic organizers to help sequence information for effective communication.
- Model brainstorming for generation of ideas.

- Explicitly teach about genres, and writing to an audience.
- Present models of good writing with guidance in determining why the writing was effective for its purpose.

General Social/Emotional Accommodations for Cognitive Functions

- Provide individualized educational program/instruction.
- Apply age and grade-level expectations with flexibility.
- Establish consistent and predictable daily routine.
- Allow preview of and gradual exposure to new activities, teachers, classes, etc.
- Use individually developed social stories.

If Verbal Comprehension Is a Relative Strength

- Talk the child through a stressful situation.
- Preview new situations with a conversation.
- Use metaphors and stories to provide context for emotional and social experiences.

If Perceptual Reasoning Is a Relative Strength

- Use visuals and manipulatives to explain social situations and emotional experiences.

Sources: Thompson (1998), College Committee on Disability Issues (2008), and Seaman (2014).

Addressing Cognitive Functions

The following section presents information on specific interventions and activities that can be used in a classroom or home environment to support an individual with various cognitive vulnerabilities. Interventions geared toward groups and individuals will be presented. This includes interventions and activities developed to foster social/emotional development and support academics. Modifying the environment of a classroom or school can also support the needs of individuals.

While these interventions and activities are designed to be ready to implement, it is important to consider the specific needs of individuals or the specific presentation of a group. Tailoring the activities to specific abilities and interests increases the motivation of the individual to participate and experience success.

In addition to planning specific activities, creating an environment that supports the individual's cognitive profile is critical. This can make assimilating information from the environment less stressful and more accessible. Possible environmental adaptations are also suggested. While directly addressing cognitive strengths and vulnerabilities through specific activities, interventions, and environmental alteration, the individual may also benefit from receiving services that are outside the purview of the classroom, such as speech and language therapy, physical therapy, individual psychotherapy, tutoring, and occupational therapy. Potential services will be listed as well. Whenever possible, it is helpful to have access to the individual who is providing the service to promote collaboration, discuss ongoing issues and interventions, and integrate the treatment the child is receiving into the classroom environment. For example, the integration of a sensory diet into the classroom might be indicated.

Verbal Comprehension Interventions and Activities

SOCIAL/EMOTIONAL

Verbal comprehension plays a role in the interactions we have with other people. It relates to the comprehension of words, ability to infer meaning, and use of language to navigate a social situation. Individuals with weak verbal comprehension skills may struggle to understand metaphors and similes or adapt their language to their intended audience. They tend to play alone at recess, play with younger children, shadow the activities of others, or disrupt play when they attempt to join in (Fujiki et al., 1999). Connections between verbal skills and difficulty regulating behavior have been established. For example, parents have reported that they find their children who have language difficulties more difficult to manage compared to typically developing siblings (Law & Garret, 2004). Benner, Nelson, and Epstein reviewed several studies in which children were identified with emotional and behavioral issues (2002). It was found that 71% of the children also experienced clinically significant language difficulties.

It has been shown that participation in language-based programs in which students role-play social situations can effectively reduce disruptive behavior (Hill & Coufal, 2005). Developing activities that encourage the integration of language into their daily experiences is also helpful. One way to do this is to develop structured predictable activities that encourage the students to share about their day. There are numerous language-based social skills development curricula available as well.

Games that Promote Verbal Reasoning Development

Crossword puzzles; anagrams; code-breakers; word searches; Scrabble; Hangman; Apples to Apples; Guess Who?; Headbandz; Bananagrams; Buzzword; Scattergories; I Spy; Magnetic Poetry; Spot It!; Slamwich; Go Fish; Boggle; and Story Cubes.

ACADEMIC

Reading Verbal comprehension is important to the development of reading skills in many ways. This cognitive skill integrates vocabulary development, basic context, and cultural life experiences for the reader to draw upon and generalize (Flanagan et al., 2002). To support the development of reading skills, engage the students in pre-reading activities such as previewing vocabulary by asking them what they already know and what they want to know and asking them to make predictions in a story.

- Teach the use of the dictionary and thesaurus.
- Have students read out loud to each other and encourage questions and discussion.
- Discuss differences and similarities between two things.

Math – Students who struggle with verbal comprehension may struggle with various mathematical skills. They may be confused about mathematical terminology, have difficulty following verbal directions, and have weak skills for monitoring steps of complex calculations (Garnett, 1998). Comprehension of word problems can also be difficult (Flanagan et al., 2002). Asking children to "play teacher" and explain concepts to their peers encourages the use of math vocabulary and ensures their understanding of the concepts. Asking the students to verbalize each step of a math problem can also strengthen verbal math skills.

ENVIRONMENTAL CONSIDERATIONS

- Develop a word wall that displays current vocabulary words.
- Label various items in the environment.
- Provide a literacy-rich environment with books of various reading levels. Be sure to include books that appeal to interests of individuals and the group and which correlate to current lesson plans.

Perceptual Reasoning Interventions and Activities

Developing interventions and activities for individuals relies on a few overarching concepts that will allow the interventions to be more accessible or successful. Planning activities that engage multiple sensory modalities, such as auditory or tactile senses, can provide experiential feedback that supports neural development (S. W. Anderson, 2002).

SOCIAL/EMOTIONAL

Individuals who struggle with perceptual skills may have difficulty with understanding non-verbal behavior, gestures, and facial expressions of other people (Forrest, 2007). Intervention can include game-like or play-like activities that foster perceptual development. Another method is participation in activities that directly teach the ability to read and understand the behavior of others and how to respond. A combination of both approaches, depending on the needs of individuals or the skill set of a group, can be utilized. It is important to keep in mind that body language is often rooted in cultural experiences and exposure. When teaching non-verbal cues, it is important to remember different cultures have different cues.

Games that Promote Perceptual Development

Simon Says; hidden pictures (such as Where's Waldo?); mazes; connect the dots; puzzles; visual memory games; matching games and mimicking/copying games; rhyming games; dominoes; card games; dice games; Jenga; Battleship; Connect Four; Spot It!; Uno; chess; checkers; Mousetrap; Lego; marble run games; building blocks; Set; Rush Hour; Tangrams; Pick-Up Sticks; Bingo; and Blokus.

Studies have found that participating in groups designed to specifically address social perception deficits can lead to improvements in social-competence skills (Guli, 2005; Glass et al., 2000). Children participated in activities adapted from drama and theatre classes in order to improve perception and interpretation of emotions and response to others' behavior. Post participation, individuals displayed fewer solitary behaviors and spent more time in positive social interactions.

Another modality for creative social/emotional development is the use of art. It can be helpful to use art to foster skills related to reading facial expressions and understanding gestures and learn how emotions are portrayed. When using art in this context, it is important to clarify with the students the difference between the use of art for pure expression versus the attempt to make an image representational. This is different from art class, where they learn specific skills and techniques.

In addition to participating in playful and creative activities that foster social understanding and interaction, specific instruction can be provided to individuals who have difficulty in this area. There are numerous evidence-based programs that have been developed that teach non-verbal social skills. These curriculum-based programs utilize various strategies.

ACADEMIC

Reading – Perceptual reasoning and vision systems play a complex role in the acquisition of reading skills. This functional domain is implicit in the development of shape and letter recognition, distinguishing words anywhere on a page even when presented in different fonts and sizes, and differentiation between shapes and lines in the environment and letters. Perceptual reasoning also plays a role in understanding the association between lower-case and upper-case letters (Dehaene, 2009). Uta Frith developed three stages that postulate how vision impacts reading development (1985). First, the child recognizes words as though they are objects and not words. Then the child develops an association between how letters and words look and the sounds paired with them. Finally, a vast lexicon of visual units develops. Intervention can take place at any one of these stages. The more senses and real-world experiences students have with different letters and words, the more likely they are to recognize letters and words and make important associations. Engaging various senses through activities can also help establish these connections. One can do so through song, dance, art, and other kinesthetic activities.

Math – Individuals with perceptual reasoning difficulties may have difficulty reading numbers and arithmetic signs, forming or copying appropriate numbers, placing numbers in columns, and consistently working from left to right (Riccio, Sullivan, & Cohen, 2010). They may also struggle with the concept of part-to-whole relationships (such as ratios or fractions). They can also struggle to understand how concepts are represented visually (various types of charts or tables, the meaning of symbols, or math operations) or how to take a three-dimensional object or space and represent it two-dimensionally (reading maps or wayfinding) (Korkman, Kirk, & Kemp, 1998). It is important to anchor these concepts to a verbal narrative that is based in repeated multi-sensory real-world experiences. These students will benefit from precise and clear verbal directions. Developing a narrative based in the experiential use of manipulatives is also important. For example, have the student hold a triangle and say, "A triangle has three sides. When we draw it, it has three connected lines" (Garnett, 1998).

ENVIRONMENTAL CONSIDERATIONS

- Free the environment of additional visual clutter. Keep the classroom organized.
- Provide visual cues using images. For example, post the daily schedule in both words and with pictures (see the Appendix, for example).
- Use visual timers to track time and set expectations. This could be done with a sand hourglass, a clock with Plexiglas that the students can draw on, or a Time Timer.
- Preview changes in the environment with the students. If furniture is going to be rearranged, inform the students before the change occurs.

Fluid Reasoning Interventions and Activities

SOCIAL/EMOTIONAL

As noted in previous sections, abstract reasoning includes various cognitive skill sets that relate to social interactions. This includes flexible thinking, pretend play, theory of mind, and making inferences. Individuals who struggle with fluid reasoning might have difficulty generalizing rules to new situations (including social rules) and difficulty with novel events, and struggle to understand the behavior and intentions of other people. In addition, individuals who struggle with abstract reasoning may find it difficult to recognize social patterns and understand subtle social cues.

Games that Promote Fluid Reasoning Development

Guess Who?; Clue; Farkel; Yahtzee; Mastermind; chess; checkers; Battleship; Sorry; Trouble; Stratego; Chinese checkers; Monopoly; Set; Rush Hour; Tower of Hanoi; Sudoku; Animal Mastermind Towers; Zendo; gin rummy; rummy; Blokus; and Risk.

ACADEMIC

Abstract reasoning is part of many academic arenas. Some general guidelines for supporting the development of abstract reasoning include:

- Solve problems with step-by-step procedures.
- Use concrete materials when learning new concepts (math, science experiments, etc.).
- Use concept mapping to illustrate relations between ideas.
- Link abstract concepts with practical and concrete examples (personally meaningful and relevant).
- Create "troubleshooting" guides to help remember how typical problems are solved (College Committee on Disability Issues, 2008).

Reading – Fluid reasoning plays a moderate role in reading development, mainly related to issues of comprehension such as drawing general conclusions from specific information (Flanagan et al., 2002).

Math – Fluid reasoning is related to mathematics at all ages and skills. For example, deciding which information in a word problem is relevant relies on fluid reasoning (Flanagan et al., 2002).

OTHER SERVICES

- Speech and language therapy,
- occupational therapy,
- individual psychotherapy, and
- tutoring or small group instruction.

Chapter 2 Appendix: Cognitive Interventions

Verbal Comprehension

GROUP STORY TIME

Goal: Creative expression using language to develop a story. Foster verbal connections between students.

Materials: Story-prompt games such as Story Cubes or Tell Tale cards. Paper and pencil.

Directions: "We are going to use these cards (or dice) to write a story as a group. Every person will have at least one turn. When it is your turn, you will pick a card from the pile and make up a very short story about the card. It will only be a few sentences long. When your turn is over, put the card in the middle of the table. Then the next person will pick a card and use that picture to add the next step to the story. Whoever starts the story must make it a beginning and whoever ends the story must make sure that the story is over. I will write down the story as we go so we can all remember it."

Adaptations:

- Allow individuals to develop their own stories based on a few cards.
- Make cards that reflect the interests of individuals or the group.
- After the story is complete, ask the students to draw a scene from the story.
- Develop the story orally without pictorial supports.

Based on: Martinovitch (2005).

UNDERSTANDING IDIOMS: LANGUAGE-BASED SOCIAL SKILLS DEVELOPMENT

Goal: Develop better understanding of figurative language, specifically commonly used idioms.

Materials: *In a Pickle and Other Funny Idioms* by Marvin Terban (1983); list of common idioms (see below). Formatted book pages (see below), binders or folders for each child, pencils, markers or crayons.

Directions: "We are going to read a book that is all about how sometimes people say things that don't make sense. The things they say might have a secret or mystery meaning. We are going to learn the secret and mystery meaning. Then we are going to make our own books!"

- Read *In a Pickle and Other Funny Idioms* to the students. Explain what an idiom is.
- Present a list of idioms and their meanings.
- Have each child choose two or three idioms to illustrate.
- Repeat the book-making process for several days or until each child is more comfortable with the use of idioms.

Adaptation: If the students need more scaffolding before making the book, they can complete an additional worksheet in which idioms are matched to their meaning. This can be scaffolded by providing images alongside the meaning.

Idioms

At the drop of a hat – to do something right away very quickly.

Back to the drawing board – when something did not work, to start over and try again.

Every cloud has a silver lining – when something goes wrong, a good thing could still happen.

Feeling a bit under the weather – feeling a little sick.

Driving me up the wall – your behavior is upsetting.

The last straw – when there are too many problems happening in one day.

On the ball – when someone understands what needs to be done and is ready to do it.

See eye to eye – to agree on something.

That is a piece of cake – something was really easy to do.

Once in a blue moon – when something doesn't happen all the time, or very rarely.

Idioms Book Worksheet

Name: ______________________

Date: _______________________

Write down the idiom____

In this box, draw what it would look like.

In this box draw what it really means.

DAILY COMIC STRIP: LANGUAGE-BASED SOCIAL SKILLS DEVELOPMENT

Goal: Foster reflection and encourage language skills related to daily events. Practice sequencing events.

Materials: Comic strip template, comic strip scaffolding worksheet, colored pencils or thin markers.

Directions: "We are going to get to know each other and learn about the different things you do. We will make comic strips about your life! Think about your day yesterday [or today, depending on what time the group is happening] and think of at least three things that you did. If you can, think of three things that you did with other people. Before we make the comic strip drawings, we will get our ideas ready using this piece of paper [show the group the graphic organizer for ideas]. Once you know what you will draw and what the people in the comic strip will say, you can start working on your drawings [show the group the comic strip template]."

Adaptations:

- For students who are unfamiliar with the schema of the speech balloon, preview the concept.
- Provide a list of commonly used conversational phrases that could be integrated into the comic strip.
- Preview new or infrequently used vocabulary that could be integrated into the comic strip.
- Depending on the graphomotor skills of the individual, offer different-sized paper with larger boxes.
- At different times of the year, this can be used to discuss activities that occur in different environments. For example, after vacations, after summer vacation, in another class, on the playground or after a field trip.
- Prior to the activity, provide comic books of different reading levels.

Comic Strip Ideas

Name: ____________________

Date: ____________________

Finish the sentences by adding words or doing a quick drawing.

In the morning on__________________________ I ____________________

____.

I talked to___________________________ and we talked about__________

____.

In the afternoon on________________________ I ____________________

____.

I talked to___________________________ and we talked about__________

____.

In the evening on__________________________ I ____________________

____.

I talked to___________________________ and we talked about__________

____.

Comic Book Pages Worksheet

Name: ____________________

Date: ________________

COMPARE/CONTRAST: VENN DIAGRAMS AND THE STINKY CHEESE MAN - READING COMPREHENSION

Goal: Develop reading comprehension skills, specifically compare/contrast utilizing both verbal comprehension and perceptual reasoning. Meet requirements for teaching different reading genres.

Materials: *The Stinky Cheese Man and Other Fairly Stupid Tales* by Jon Scieszka and Lane Smith, a version of the Gingerbread Man story (for example, the one by Richard Scarry), the Stinky Cheese Man/Gingerbread Man Venn diagram worksheet (next page), pencils.

Directions: Introduce the genre of folk tales. Preview any new vocabulary words that may be in either story. If the class is comprised of older children, assure them you are aware they are too old for the story but that they need to learn about folk tales as part of school. Read both versions of the story to the class. Discuss similarities and differences between each version, taking notes on the discussion. Hand out worksheets and allow students to complete the activity as a group or independently, depending on their skill level and understanding of Venn diagrams.

Adaptations:

- Can be used to discuss the concept of a parody.
- If the students have fine motor skill difficulties, complete the activity as a group on a large piece of paper, Smart Board or other board with teacher scribing.

Name : ______________________

Date : ______________________

Gingerbread Man

Gingerbread Man
AND
Stinky Cheese Man

Stinky Cheese Man

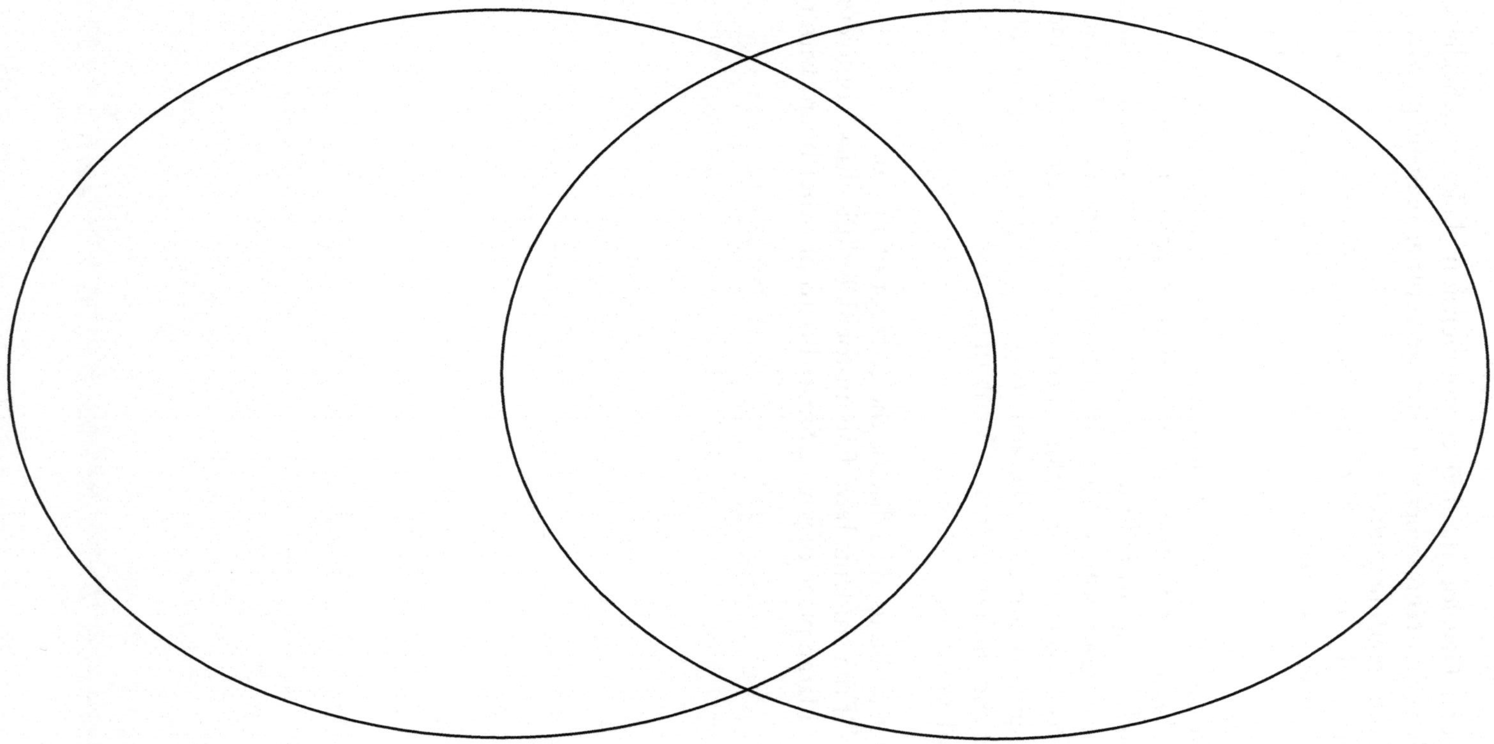

MATH VOCABULARY WORD WALL: VERBAL COMPREHENSION MATH ACTIVITY

Goal: Increase math vocabulary, support understanding, and make definitions readily accessible and applicable.

Materials: Space on the wall to post words (the word wall – developed by Cunningham and Allington, 1994) – this can be done with paper cards, sheets of paper or other classroom materials; flashlight or laser pointer.

Directions: Select content-specific math vocabulary words for the unit you are teaching. As you teach the unit, take time to define important words and highlight their presence on the word wall, adding them as you teach. Once words are posted and students are familiar with them, turn off the classroom lights and hand out flashlights or laser pointers. Make the statement, "The definition of ______ is . . ." Ask the group or individuals to shine their light on the matching word. Be sure to give time for the group to think about the answer.

Perceptual Reasoning

FEELINGS CHARADES: DRAMA INTERVENTIONS

Goal: Embody or act out a variety of feelings. Guess what feelings are being acted out.

Materials: Cards with different feelings written on them and a corresponding drawing (smiley face, sad face, etc.), chairs for all the students to sit in, a space large enough for one person to move around safely.

Directions: "We are going to play a guessing game. Each person will get a chance to be an actor. You will pick a card from this pile and act out the feeling that is on it. If you need help knowing how to act it out, you can ask. The kids in the audience will raise their hands and try to guess what feeling you are acting out."

Adaptation: Two students can act out the feeling together.

BUS STOP GAME: IMPROVISATION DRAMA INTERVENTION

This game is intended to help students engage with people and portray emotions, and to allow the audience to guess what feelings are being acted out. Prior to playing this game, it may be helpful to play Feelings Charades first.

Goal: Engage with each other, pretending to be various characters with specific emotions.

Materials: Two chairs, character cards – each card has a character that the student might be familiar with (sad person, happy person, cranky/mad person, or specific characters from TV shows or movies the students like), conversation-starter cards (each card has a line on it to help the student engage the person who is waiting; for example, "Hi there, it is really hot today, huh?" or "I really like the shirt that you're wearing.").

Directions: "We are going to play a game. We will pretend that these two chairs are a bench at a bus stop. We will be waiting for a bus. One person will sit on the 'bench' and pretend to be someone. The second person will walk up to them and start a conversation. They will also pretend to be someone. You can make up your own character or pick one from these character cards. If you want help knowing how to start a conversation with the person sitting on the bench, you can use one of these conversation-starter cards. The people in the audience will raise their hands and guess what feelings your character has or who the character is. The scene ends when the first person leaves to get on the bus. Then a new person will enter the scene and we can guess who they are."

Adaptations:

- Integrate props.
- Depending on the skill level of the students and their experience with this game, do not provide cards and allow them to develop their own characters.
- Add three people to the interaction instead of two.

SOCIAL ROLE-PLAY: DRAMA INTERVENTION

Goal: Create common social situations that the students may encounter. Allow for individual and group problem-solving. Practice social skills in a safe, predictable, and less stressful environment.

Materials: Chairs and table, cards with various social situations and common problems that may occur (birthday party without likable food, receiving a non-preferred gift, attending a wedding, going shopping and not getting a desired object, being bored at dinner, trying to integrate into a group of children playing at recess, playing games/activities that are undesirable, etc.). Make the problematic social situation age-appropriate and contextualized to the lives of the students.

Directions: "We are going to play a game where we pretend we are going somewhere or doing something where a problem can happen. We will pick a card that tells the story of where we are going and what the problem is. As a group, we will decide how many actors we need and what their roles are. We will talk about ways to solve the problem, things that people can say and how the story will end. Once we have a plan, we will act it out. People in the audience can raise their hands and, when they are called on, make a new suggestion if the plan we made isn't working out."

Adaptations:

- Allow students to generate a list of situations they have experienced or are worried about experiencing.
- Integrate props.

TEAM DRAWING: ART INTERVENTION

Goal: Foster social connections without the use of words. Regulate behavior in relationship to another person.

Materials: 8.5 x 11 inch paper (size of paper can be altered), markers.

Directions: "You are going to work with a partner to make a drawing. You will be taking turns to make one image. Decide who will take the first turn. That person chooses a colored marker and makes a small line, dot, or shape. Once they have finished, the other person will look at what their friend drew, pick another color, and add a small line, dot, or shape. You will keep taking turns until you decide together that the drawing is done. The drawing might end up looking like a bunch of lines, dots, or shapes or it could end up looking like animals, a place, people, or whatever you like. Before you start, ask your partner if it is okay for you to draw over something they have made or if you should only draw close to it."

Adaptations:

- This activity can be done in the span of 30 minutes. If there is more time, students can take turns making images with other partners.
- Start with a relatively small piece of paper until the students are accustomed to the concept. Using larger pieces of paper or other drawing media can change or enhance the experience.
- When working with children who have sensory sensitivities, be aware that chalk or pastels can make them uncomfortable.
- Expand to include three artists per piece of paper, depending on the size of the paper.
- Do the activity as a sidewalk drawing. Make sure to indicate the space allotted for each drawing pair.

Based on: Hinz (2009).

FEELINGS COLLAGE: ART INTERVENTION

Goals: Identify facial expressions in a non-stressful environment.

Materials: 11 × 14 inch mixed-media paper, a box of magazine clippings or old magazines, glue sticks, markers. Choose a feeling that is relatively easy to identify (such as happy, sad, or mad). It is best to start with a feeling that does not evoke a potentially negative experience.

Directions: "We are going to make a collage [or a couple of collages] that help us understand what faces look like when someone is having a feeling. There are all these pictures from magazines. You will get a pile of pictures. Please sort through your pile and find all the faces that look happy. Take the pictures of happy faces and glue them to your piece of paper. Once you have found enough happy faces to fill up the paper, decorate the paper using your markers."

Adaptations:

- Make several collages that portray different facial expressions.
- Divide the piece of paper into equal sections. Each section can contain a different feeling. Make sure the paper isn't visually overwhelming.
- Make a feelings box: each side of the box is covered in magazine clippings that portray facial expressions or different feelings.
- Offer other materials that can be used to decorate the collage, such as stickers (ones that might display facial expressions; for example, happy faces or emojis), gem stones, glitter, or paint.
- Limit material if the students are easily overwhelmed.

Body Language Worksheet

People use their bodies to tell us what they are thinking and feeling. This is called body language. Watching how they are using their bodies can give us important clues.

Look at the list of types of body language and write down what you think the body language means. Use the list of ideas or make your own.

Looking at you with a big smile ______________________________

Walking toward you with their arms open wide________________

Rolling eyes ____

Shrugging shoulders____

Slumping in a chair____

Nodding when someone is talking ____________________________

Waving their hands in the air_________________________________

Sitting or standing with arms crossed_________________________

Shaking their head when someone is talking__________________

Bored

Tired

Angry

Happy

Agrees with you

Does not agree with you

Excited

Does not know what to say

Frustrated

Perceptual Reasoning

RECOGNIZING MATHEMATICAL SYMBOLS: PERCEPTUAL REASONING SUPPORT

Goal: Promote understanding/recognition of mathematical symbols and how they represent real-world concepts.

Materials: Leaves, sticks, rocks, or any item that has been collected from the playground or outdoor space – if the students are not interested in nature, have them collect marbles, counting bears, or other objects that have been hidden around the classroom; two flash cards, one with an addition symbol and the other with a subtraction symbol.

Directions: Have the students collect items and put them in a large pile or bucket. Dump or place several of the items onto the table or floor and have the group count the number of items aloud as a chorus. Ask the group, "What if we put more ______ into our pile? How many would we have then?" Add the number of items to the pile, asking the students to count along in chorus. As a group, "What if we take away _____ (number) of the _______? How many would we have then?" Have the students count along as you subtract items. Continue this activity until students understand the concepts of addition and subtraction. Substitute the words "addition" and "subtraction" for "put more in" and "take away from." When they are comfortable using ***addition*** and ***subtraction***, display each symbol. Explain that they represent adding and subtracting. Continue with the activity, but this time hold up the symbol each time items are added to or removed from the pile. Allow the students to hold up symbols as well.

Adaptations:

- Invite students to determine the number of items added or subtracted to the pile. They can physically move the items themselves, temporarily acting as the group leader.
- Adapt this activity for other mathematical symbols, including multiplication, division, equal sign (=) and more than/less than signs (>, <).

Based on: Frye et al., 2005.

FRACTIONS LESSON PLAN: REAL-WORLD PART-TO-WHOLE RELATIONSHIPS

Goal: Divide objects into halves. Differentiate between wholes and halves.

Materials: Several apples, oranges, pears, etc.; a knife for slicing the fruit; play dough (can be homemade or make it with the students if appropriate); worksheets with images of the fruit cut into pieces.

Directions: Show the students two apples. Ask, "If there were two kids who wanted an apple, how many apples would each kid get?" Once they understand each child would get one apple, put an apple away. Now state, "I have one apple. Two kids want some apple. How many apples would each kid get? How can I make it fair?" Demonstrate slicing the apple in half. Verbally state, "I cannot give each child a whole apple. They can only have part of an apple. Each child will get half of an apple. This is what half of an apple looks like." Ask the kids if one is bigger than the other. Ask them if splitting the apple this way feels fair. Hand out the play dough and ask the children to make various shapes with the dough (providing visual cues on what the shapes should look like). Using play dough tools, instruct the students to divide each shape in half. Be sure to narrate the process. Once they have completed dividing several shapes, clean up the play dough and have them complete a simple fractions worksheet.

Adaptation:

- Use this activity to describe fourths, eighths and so on.

Fluid Reasoning

PREVIEW NEW SOCIAL SITUATIONS/ENVIRONMENT: SWIMMING POOL EXAMPLE

Goal: Help a child feel comfortable and confident in new social situations or environments. This can be done for many social activities (parties, weddings, funerals, eating out in restaurants, shopping trips, vacations, etc.) and environments. This example focuses on swimming pools because they can be an overwhelming sensory experience.

Material: Make a small photo album with pictures of common environmental items that would be found at a pool. If you can use the actual pool, that is best. Be sure to include the shallow end, the deep end, ladders and steps, diving boards, benches and chairs, and any toys that might be available. Write out the "Rules of the Pool." If the child is young or struggles with verbal comprehension, include simple images beside each rule. Have the bathing suit, towels, and other pool equipment you are planning to use.

Direction: Explain to the child that you will be doing something new together. Present the idea of going to a swimming pool and all of the fun things that can happen at the pool. Let the child know what behaviors are expected of them and that general safety rules apply at the pool. Show them the pictures of the swimming pool and explain the image. Show them the "Rules of the Pool" and set clear expectations. Show them the swimsuit they will use. If you plan to change at the pool changing rooms, give them step-by-step directions for the process both before and after swimming. It may be best to chunk this information over a couple of days. Let the child know what their options are if they start to feel overwhelmed or get upset. Establish an area for taking breaks and provide soothing activities specific to the individual. Giving them these options ahead of time helps develop appropriate coping skills. If possible and depending on the needs of the individual, call the swimming pool and ask if they have special needs services available.

Adaptations:

- Make this appropriate to the child's developmental level and area of interests, the activity, and the environment.
- Be sure to use clear and concise language and preview new words if the child also struggles with verbal comprehension. If it is a strength, be sure to avoid infantilizing the child.

CAUSE-AND-EFFECT IN SOCIAL SITUATIONS

Goal: Help students recognize cause-and-effect relationships in social interactions. This allows them to make sense of the behaviors and reactions of other people. Reading comprehension development can also be fostered through this activity.

Materials: The books *If You Give a Mouse a Cookie*, *If You Give a Moose a Muffin*, *If You Give a Pig a Pancake* and *If You Give a Cat a Cupcake* by Laura Numeroff and illustrated by Felicia Bond; white board, chalk board, or Smart Board; paper, pencil, or individual white boards and markers.

Directions: Start the activity with two sentences on the board that display cause-and-effect. For example:

- The children stayed inside and played board games during recess.
- It was raining outside during recess time.

Explain that something happens first and that people make a choice or have a reaction to the first thing. Ask the group what happened first in these two sentences. Provide a few more examples that are self-referential for the group and that involve their interests. Ask the kids to make their own cause-and-effect sentences, either writing or drawing them on paper or white boards. Read the book *If You Give a Mouse a Cookie*, instructing the students to raise their hands and point out cause-and-effect within the book as you read it aloud. Tell the students that all the books will be available for them to read during break times.

Adaptations:

- Have the students choose one of their favorite animals and write their own version of the *If You Give a . . .* books.
- Have the students write and act out skits that display cause-and-effect in social relationships.
- Have the students write comic strips with cause-and-effect social situations.

PREVIEW READING COMPREHENSION PASSAGE

Goal: Improve student comprehension of a passage by promoting attention to specific information.

Materials: A reading passage that is appropriate to grade level and curriculum requirements, a list of specific vocabulary words within the passage, a list of comprehension questions specific to the passage.

Directions: Prior to reading the passage, the teacher previews new vocabulary words. The teacher also presents comprehension questions, both orally and in written format. After reading the passage, the teacher summarizes it. The students are then asked to read the passage and locate answers to each question.

RELEVANT VS. IRRELEVANT INFORMATION: MATH PROBLEM-SOLVING

Goal: Help students discern between irrelevant and relevant information in a word problem. This activity assumes they know how to add and subtract.

Materials: Relevant vs. Irrelevant Information worksheet, pencils, M&M's, Skittles, truck stickers, a small plastic horse toy (the candy, stickers, or other items do not need to be these specific materials; develop individualized worksheets that relate to the interests of the students in the class and bring matching manipulatives to the lesson).

Directions: Preview the words "relevant" and "irrelevant," including them in a math vocabulary word wall. They can be defined as:

Relevant: Information that you need.

Irrelevant: Information you do not need even if it is interesting.

Tell the class, "We are going to work as a group to solve a couple of word problems. We are going to be detectives while we do this! The word problems have extra information in them and we need to decide what information is important. Important information is relevant. Information we do not need is irrelevant. We will read the problem together. I will show you what the problem is using these things [point at candies, stickers, and toys]. You will help me decide what question I am trying to answer and what information is extra. We will fill out these charts to help us." Pass out worksheets. As you read the first problem, make sure you have 20 M&M's and act out the problem as you read it. Point at the Skittles. Do the same for the word problem with stickers.

Adaptations:

- For students with graphomotor issues, allow them to abbreviate "relevant" as "R" and "irrelevant" as "I."
- Once the worksheet is complete, encourage the students to make their own word problems about themselves that have extra information in them. They can select items from the classroom to demonstrate the word problems to their peers.
- Be sure to develop word problems that match the interests and experiences of students in your classroom. This type of strategy can be used for more word problems as concepts become increasingly complex and/or abstract.

Relevant vs. Irrelevant Information

Name: ____________________

Date: ____________________

Melissa has 20 M&M's. She really likes Skittles. She gives 6 M&M's to Thomas. How many M&M's does Melissa have left?

What question are you trying to answer? ____________________________

Information	*Relevant or Irrelevant?*

What is the answer to the question? ________________________________

Henry has 15 truck stickers. His friend Keisha gives him 7 more stickers. Keisha has 4 horses. How many truck stickers does Henry have now?

What questions are you trying to answer? ______________________

Information	*Relevant or Irrelevant?*

What is the answer to the question? ______________________

–3–

Executive Functioning Interventions

Introduction

The term "executive functions" (EFs) refers to a constellation of skills that allow to set a goal and maintain behavior to achieve it (Luria, 1966). As was discussed regarding cognition, to a certain extent, these skills are circumscribed by the ways in which we are able to measure executive functioning abilities. The following are subdomains of EFs that were treated in more depth in our previous publication and which lend themselves to a variety of measurement tools (Reinstein & Burau, 2014). For our current purposes, these categories can be subsumed under three major domains: Thinking Skills, Impulse Control, and Working Memory.

Thinking Skills

- ***Concept Generation/Formation***: distinguish relevant information, follow rules, and apply knowledge base to new situations.
- ***Plan, Organize, Reason, and Problem Solve***: organize materials, sequence steps, make decisions based on objective information, make inferences, weigh priorities, and form conclusions.
- ***Shift Set/Perseverate***: perform a task and switch to another as appropriate (shift set)/ repeat a behavior when it is maladaptive (perseverate). Cognitive flexibility allows one to transition between tasks and avoid perseveration.

- ***Attention***: bring one's focus onto a limited number of stimuli or tasks at one time and sustain it over a period.
- ***Fluency***: spontaneously react and generate new responses to environmental cues or stimuli in a timely manner.

Impulse Control

- ***Inhibition/Distractibility***: filter out (inhibit a focus on) irrelevant internal or external information (distractions) as a means to sustain attention.
- ***Behavioral and Emotional Regulation***: attend, inhibit inappropriate responding, and manage impulsivity during an emotional response.
- ***Use of Feedback/Self-Monitoring***: monitor one's actions while performing a task in order to derive feedback about accuracy or errors, manage time, and make decisions.

Working Memory

- ***Working Memory***: hold bits of information in one's head and perform operations on that information. For auditory working memory, the phonological loop; for visuospatial working memory, the visuospatial sketchpad.

Observing Executive Functions

EFs are skills we utilize for a variety of activities throughout the day. Developing observational skills in these settings can help translate assessment results into real-world interventions. The following list of questions can be used while observing a child to help identify issues or strengths within EFs.

General Executive Function Observations

Do they often complain of getting bored despite not finishing work or displaying mastery?

Do they quickly fatigue or lose interest? What is their stamina for different activities?

Do they spend too much time on an assignment?

Do they benefit from having extra time to develop responses to questions?

Are they often losing important items? Forgetting essential materials?

Do they often lose items during transitions?

Do transitions require extra time or excessive redirection?

Despite demonstrating knowledge of math concepts, are they unable to identify solutions to problems?

Do they struggle with new social situations or large social events?

Are transitions overwhelming or confusing?

Working Memory

Do they struggle with multi-step directions?

If you ask them to complete three tasks, can they do it without reminders?

Do they struggle to complete simple math operations in their head?

Do they forget what they were going to say when called on in class?

Do they require frequent reminders and repetition?

Do they forget what they were doing?

Do they have trouble remembering information for a few seconds?

Do they have difficulty thinking and retaining information at the same time?

Do they struggle to remember what they just saw?

Do they lose their place when counting?

Do they struggle to organize information while writing?

When in the middle of an activity, do they forget how to complete it?

Do they struggle with mental arithmetic?

When writing, does the good use of reasoning or visuospatial abilities deteriorate as writing progresses?

Do they complain that once they start writing they forget what they were writing about?

Do they have a low frustration tolerance?

Do they infrequently participate in classroom discussion?

Impulse Control

Do they display difficulty with getting started on activities, zoning out, sustaining interest, or using developed skills consistently?

Despite having adequate ideas and language representation, is their written production limited or avoided?

Do they resist using pencils or display an awkward grasp?

Do they quickly fatigue during writing activities?

Do they notice when there are inaccuracies, poor wording, poor punctuation, and misspelling?

Do they understand if they have done an assignment correctly?

Do they reverse numbers or incorrectly sequence them? Do they miss steps in math problems or use the wrong operational sign?

Despite having adequate handwriting skills, is their writing illegible or disorganized?

When translating information from one source to another, do they struggle to do it accurately?

During conversation, do they often introduce tangential topics?

Do they often interrupt or have difficulty waiting to speak? Once it is their turn to speak, have they forgotten what they were going to say?

Thinking Skills

When reading, do they tend to make quick but inaccurate offerings for individual words with no recognition of error? The words may start with a similar visual configuration or same letter combination.

Do they mispronounce words they have been able to previously recognize by sight and correctly pronounce? Or indicate they don't know the meaning of a word they previously knew?

Do they draw a blank on math problems they were previously able to solve?

Do they struggle to apply decoding skills when reading sentences and passages they have learned to correctly decode?

When reading nonsense words, do they substitute real sight-words instead of decoding? Is their word, sentence, or passage reading rate not commensurate with the rate demonstrated during fluency instruction?

Do they struggle with making connections between what they already know and what they are currently reading?

When asked questions about a passage they just read, do they need to re-read the passage in order to answer the questions?

When writing, do they appear resistant to generating topic ideas or accepting ideas from an outside source? Once an idea is generated, do they quickly forget it?

Is their written text overly simplistic despite having strong knowledge, adequate language, and visuospatial reasoning skills?

Do they spell words correctly in one context, but when generalizing to another context spell words incorrectly?

Are well-known mathematical calculations applied incorrectly or out of sequence?

When conversation topics or play activities have moved to a new theme, can they change themes, or do they persist on the old topic/activity?

Do they struggle to understand what other people might be thinking?

Sources: Dehn, 2012; McCloskey et al., 2014; Gathercole et al., 2006.

Observation and Development of Executive Functions

Table 3.1 highlights the developmental trajectories of the three subdomains of executive functioning skills and the assessment tools used to measure them at various ages. While we have separated the subdomains of executive functioning for our purposes, this is an artificial distinction that is made because of the current limitations on the manner in which aspects of executive functioning are tested. Needless to say, the development of each subdomain is, to a varying degree, dependent on the emergence of another executive functioning skill. For example, the ability to assess working memory at a young age depends on the child's ability to inhibit impulsive responding (see Best & Miller, 2010). Therefore, when considering interventions, it is important to consider which subtests of the following assessment tools have been used to identify and evaluate a specific executive functioning subdomain. For further details, see Reinstein and Burau (2014).

Developing Accommodations and Interventions

Once a child's strengths and vulnerabilities in the EFs have been identified through observation and assessment, accommodations and interventions can be developed. The following sections begin to indicate specific types of interventions. Always individualize the intervention and consider the emotional state of the child. To that end, both academic and social/emotional interventions and accommodations will be presented. Furthermore, it is important to remember that all of the following accommodations and strategies are best implemented within the context of a holding environment (Winnicott, 1965) that has a foundation based in the relationship formed between the teacher or specialist and the child.

General Academic Accommodations and Strategies

The following list of accommodations and strategies can be implemented in the classroom. Some of these accommodations can be included in an IEP or 504 plan.

- Provide (color-coded) checklist for tasks.
- Reduce amount of work.
- Reduce course load.
- Provide preferential seating.
- Provide visual schedule.
- Use visual reminders for supplies and materials.
- Use timers to track time.
- Provide extra time for tests/exams.
- Allow access to a computer and/or organization software for tests.
- Provide copies of class notes.
- Provide structure and routines.
- Rehearse getting from place to place, pointing out significant markers.
- Provide parents with daily schedule for preview and rehearsal.
- Frequently monitor student's performance and redirect as necessary.
- Develop a therapeutic behavioral modification plan.

TABLE 3.1 Executive Function Development

Age	*Thinking Skills*	*Impulse Control*	*Working Memory*	*Assessments*
3–5 years	• Shift between two response sets within the context of a story • Understand and apply different rules in different contexts • Perform a simple self-help task (brush teeth) • Straighten up bedroom with help	• Beginning around four years, delay immediate gratification • Reduction of perseveration in conflict tasks • Improved ability to hold a posture in the face of distractions • By four years, success on both simple and complex inhibition tasks	• Toddlers keep two different rules in mind • Ability to run simple errands (get boots from closet)	• Bayley-III • WPPSI-IV • SB-5 • WJ-IV • K-ABC-II
5–6 years	• Use feedback from a previous task to shift set using novel information • Straighten up bedroom • Bring papers to and from school • Decide how to spend money	• Impulse control continues to improve due to increased ability to override hardwired responses • Follow safety rules	• Ability to perform more complex tasks that require the coordination of WM subcomponents • Complete errands with two- to three-step directions	• WPPSI-IV • SB-5 • WJ-IV • K-ABC-II

6–12 years	• Increased flexible thinking allows for setting goals and changing strategies • Increased ability to adapt to changing rules • Able to bring books, assignments to and from school • Keep track of belongings away from home • Complete homework assignments • Plan simple projects	• Ability to ignore unimportant visual information improves • Save money for desired objects rather than spend it right away • Inhibit/self-regulate behavior when teacher is not present	• Ability to search for objects in three different locations matures by age 6 • Ability to run more complex errands (time delay or greater distance)	• WPPSI-IV (up to 7:7 years) • SB-5 • WJ-IV • K-ABC-II • WISC-V • D-KEFS
13–18 years	• Shifting ability reaches adult levels at about 15 • Improved ability to shift focus and adapt to changes in rules • Increased control over thinking skills • Able to help with chores at home • Use system for organizing schoolwork • Follow complex school schedule • Plan and carry out long-term projects • Plan time (after-school activities, homework, etc.)	• Increased ability to focus attention and ignore irrelevant information • Inhibit rule-breaking in absence of authority • Inhibit reckless and dangerous behaviors	• Ability to retain main points of lecture while taking notes • Ability to search for objects in four locations matures and for up to eight locations continues to mature into adulthood	• SB-5 • WJ-IV • K-ABC-2 • WISC-V (up to 16:11 years) • D-KEFS

Sources: Anderson (2015); Best & Miller (2010); Dawson & Guare (2010).

Working Memory General Accommodations

- Provide step-by-step guidelines and procedures.
- Allow access to multi-sensory lessons and study materials.
- Provide explicit instruction on mnemonics (listing, chunking, imagining, drawing, mapping, devising acronyms and associations).
- Frequently drill and review material (cue cards, writing out key information, mind maps, etc.).
- Write out, provide visuals, or tape-record multi-step directions.
- Inform students and parents of test dates well in advance.
- Provide extended testing time.
- Do not require student to take notes.
- Utilize recognition testing such as providing a word bank.
- Provide review sheets in the same format as the test.
- Teach rehearsal strategies.
- Use word retrieval prompts.

Working Memory Reading Accommodations

- Pre-read textbook material before lectures.
- Provide list of high-frequency words.
- Provide remediation that increases phonological awareness.
- Assist in highlighting key words in textbook.
- Circle vocabulary words on worksheets.

Working Memory Math Accommodations

- Allow access to formula sheets during tests.
- Allow use of manipulatives.

Working Memory Writing Accommodations

- Provide list of frequent errors to support editing.
- Provide list of high-frequency words.
- Allow use of recorder for brainstorming.

Impulse Control General Accommodations

- Anticipate and rehearse plans to cope with complex situations.
- Reinforce on-task behavior.
- Reduce distractions in environment and for assignments and tests.
- Shorten duration of tasks.
- Reduce assignment length.
- Break assignments into small manageable chunks.
- Remind student of time.
- Use timer to define designated work times.
- Reward/praise student for getting work done in the designated time.

- Provide recording of lectures.
- Allow frequent breaks during class and testing.
- Allow program selection in area of interest.
- Alternate between activities and quiet study sessions.
- Provide visual cues that define personal space (use painter's tape on the floor).
- Develop private cue for staying on task.
- Have parents sign homework.
- Avoid open-concept classrooms.
- Provide movement breaks.
- Allow student to stand during work times.

Impulse Control Reading Accommodations

- Select texts with less on page.
- Assign shorter reading passages.
- Avoid oral reading.

Impulse Control Math Accommodations

- Highlight operation signs for math calculations.
- Use handouts with clear step-by-step directions.
- Allow use of calculator for assignments in class, homework, and on tests when appropriate.
- Decrease number of math problems on page or in assignment.
- Use graph paper to line up numbers correctly.
- Frequently check work for accuracy.
- Use individual dry erase boards.

Impulse Control Writing Accommodations

- Accept non-written forms of reports (displays, oral presentation projects, etc.).
- Allow use of assistive writing technology and/or voice-to-text software.
- Test knowledge of grammar, sentence structure, etc., with multiple-choice or fill-in-the-blank questions.
- Break writing assignments into small manageable chunks.
- Avoid assigning large quantities of written work.
- Do not penalize poor handwriting if visual-motor deficits are present.

Thinking Skills General Accommodations

- Check the notebook/planner daily.
- Color-code notebooks and folders by subject.
- Require an assignment notebook or banner.
- Provide extra time for assignments when negotiated in advance.
- Record lectures.
- Provide learning strategies training.

- Allow frequent breaks in class and during test-taking.
- Allow program selection in area of interest.
- Alternate between active and quiet study sessions.
- Allow access to manipulative materials.
- Teach metacognitive skills.
- Reinforce flexible thinking and behavior with praise.
- Use checklists.
- Preview transitions.
- Clearly identify new topics.
- Provide visual cues for shifting topics.
- Provide multi-sensory cueing.

Consider similar accommodations to those for impulse control.

Thinking Skills Reading Accommodations

- Use graphic organizers.

Thinking Skills Math Accommodations

- Highlight operational signs for calculations.

Thinking Skills Writing Accommodations

- Allow access to word processor and/portable keyboard.
- Allow access to text-to-speech software with highlighting features.
- Allow use of editing software with read-back features.

General Social/Emotional Accommodations for Executive Functions

- Provide personal space.
- Apply age- and grade-level expectations with flexibility.
- Praise compliant behavior.
- Ignore minor, inappropriate behavior.
- Avoid verbal corrections in front of entire classroom.
- Provide immediate feedback.
- Provide small groups and social skills training.
- Use social stories and narratives.
- Explicitly teach coping strategies (breathing exercises, counting backwards, etc.).
- Provide scripts for appropriate language/behaviors.
- Utilize positive reinforcement plan.
- Introduce self-monitoring strategies (feelings thermometer/rating scale, etc.).

Sources: Thomason, 1998; Morel & Berzins, 2003; Dehn, 2014; Rief, 2005; and Zeigler Dendy, 2011.

Addressing Executive Functions

The following section presents information on specific interventions and activities that can be used in a classroom or home environment to support an individual with EF vulnerabilities. This includes interventions and activities developed to foster social/emotional development and support academics. Modifying the environment of a classroom or school can also support the needs of individuals. Tailoring the activities to specific abilities and interests increases the motivation of the individual to participate and experience success.

In addition to planning specific activities, developing an environment that supports the individual's EFs is critical. Whenever possible, it is helpful to have access to the individuals who are providing outside services to promote collaboration, discuss ongoing issues and interventions, and integrate the treatment the individual is receiving into the classroom environment. For example, strategies developed during organization tutoring could be utilized in the classroom.

General Interventions for Executive Functions

In any classroom group, it is likely one or more students will struggle with different aspects of EFs to varying degrees. The following suggestions can be utilized to support entire groups of students.

WHOLE-GROUP INTERVENTIONS

- Utilize scoring rubrics to set expectations. Depending on the needs of the group, discuss the rubric or make it into a checklist.
- Visually post the daily schedule and classroom rules. Frequently review. Provide both verbal (written words) and visual (simple images) as developmentally appropriate.
- Use verbal prompts or reminders. These can be used to acquire classroom attention ("Eyes on me," etc.), remind students what materials they need even when it seems obvious ("Get out your paper and pencil"), or help them attend to their own work ("Stay separate from your neighbor's work"). This is most effective when prompts are unique to the personality of the group; use humor or an inside joke of the classroom group.
- Design group incentive programs to encourage peer support.
- Develop group routines, particularly around transitions.

ENVIRONMENTAL CONSIDERATIONS

- Carefully consider seating. Do the students face each other? Do they need separate study spaces? Who should be placed close to the teacher? Are they near a window or open door?
- Arrange furniture so teacher has unobstructed view of all students.
- Avoid wide open spaces. Arrange furniture to break up the space in an organized and uncluttered manner.

Aside from specific teaching strategies and environmental considerations, other activities can support the development of working memory. Learning to play an instrument, participating in music classes, singing in rounds and parts, dancing, and participating in theater all rely on various EFs (self-monitoring, working memory, selective attention, cognitive flexibility, etc.). These activities can be highly motivating, encourage pro-social behaviors, and exercise EFs (Center on the Developing Child at Harvard University, 2014).

Teaching self-talk is another skill that can be taught on an individual level in order to promote awareness and self-regulation (Dawson & Guare, 2010; Ylvisaker & Feeney, 2002). Self-talk is rooted in developmental and cognitive-behavioral therapy approaches. It is the internalization of language that helps us to establish goals, understand social rules, and provide the next step. Therapists and educators can utilize this strategy to help students identify specific vulnerabilities and develop solutions. Teaching children to ask themselves these four questions is the initial step to developing strong self-talk skills:

1. "What is the problem?"
2. "What is the plan?"
3. "Am I following my plan?"
4. "How did I do?"

This can be done through direct instruction and in a playful manner. The topic of the self-talk can be specific to the student's strengths and vulnerabilities.

OTHER SERVICES

- Speech and language therapy,
- occupational therapy,
- individual or group psychotherapy/expressive therapy, and
- EF tutoring/coaching.

Working Memory

Current research provides conflicting evidence about the ability to develop working memory skills when they have been shown to be weak (Dehn, 2011; Melby-Lervag & Hulme, 2013). However, providing supports and accommodations can promote successful learning. By developing activities that reduce the amount of information a child has to mentally store while engaged in another activity (such as remembering a series of numbers or the precise wording of a complex sentence), the more likely they are to experience success and maintain motivation (Gathercole et al., 2006). To do so, be sure to:

- Ensure that the child can remember the tasks by keeping instructions brief and linguistically simple. Frequently repeat the instructions. Ask the child or classroom group to repeat them.
- Use external memory aids and manipulatives. In order to make use of these aids during more complex activities, individuals struggling with working memory issues will need practice and direct instruction.
- Make the task of locating key information easier by highlighting it or providing lists of high-frequency spelling words or new words.
- Reduce the processing load of various activities.
- Teach metacognitive skills as they relate to working memory and develop awareness around when to utilize strategies (Minear & Shah, 2006).

- Utilize verbal prompts and reminders such as naming materials required for an activity even if it is easy to assume the students know (such as paper and pencils).
- Post visual cues such as classroom rules, and review rules regularly.

Aside from providing environmental supports and accommodations for working memory, researchers have attempted to develop repetitive training exercises that improve working memory (Morrison & Chein, 2011). In order for these exercises to be effective, they must be motivating enough for the student to practice them on a regular basis, require simultaneous processing and storage, and constantly adapt so the task remains challenging. However, conflicting evidence indicates that memory training programs appear to produce short-term specific training effects that do not generalize to activities other than the training exercises (Melby-Lervag & Hulme, 2013). Therefore, these exercises should be utilized with caution, especially since they can be time-consuming and expensive.

SOCIAL/EMOTIONAL

Working memory, both auditory and visual, allows an individual to hold onto and manipulate information from the environment. This can impact an individual's social skills. Much of the research on working memory and social skills development focuses on the relationship between working memory and children diagnosed with Attention Deficit/Hyperactivity Disorder (ADHD). Children struggling with working memory but who do not meet the criteria for ADHD have different social profiles than children with ADHD. They tend to have strong social skills and pro-social behaviors (Gathercole et al., 2006). Children who meet the criteria for ADHD, and difficulty with working memory, do not alway report social difficulties, but parents and teachers often report observing social struggles (Kofler et al., 2010). In short, the connection between working memory, ADHD, and social skills development is still being explored. A 2007 study indicated that working memory plays a role in an individual's ability to rapidly interpret verbal and nonverbal social and emotional cues in other people (Phillips et al.). While this area requires more research, supporting individuals in their ability to understand social cues and reflect on their own behavior can promote social development.

Games that Promote Working Memory

Crazy Eights; Uno; Go Fish; War; matching games; card games such as hearts, spades and bridge; call-and-response songs like "BooM Chicka BooM" and "I Met a Bear"; songs and games that involve clapping and singing, such as Miss Mary Mack or Down Down Baby; and Rat-a-Tat Cat.

ACADEMIC

Reading – Deficits in this functional domain are reliably found in children who do poorly on assessments of reading comprehension. Working memory contributes directly and indirectly to the acquisition of reading skills in various ways, including word reading, phonological processing, working memory in inhibitory processes, making inferences, comprehension monitoring, and semantic work knowledge (Cain, 2006).

Math – To support the development of mental arithmetic, concrete contextual support leads to the production of more correct answers during mental math activities in 4- to 5-year-olds. In other words, encouraging students to imagine that the numbers in mental math represent familiar hypothetical toys (giving the problem meaning) improves their performance (Davis & Bamford, 1995). Many studies have supported the claim that visual spatial working memory strongly impacts developing mathematical competencies. Verbal systems of processing information have also been implicated in the role of working memory as it relates to solving mathematical problems. Studies have shown that different aspects of working memory relate to mathematics achievement at different ages and at varying levels of mathematics complexity (Bull & Espy, 2006). As a result, it is important to support both verbal and visual spatial skill development as they relate to arithmetic and to provide context. These strategies will support WM deficits.

ENVIRONMENTAL CONSIDERATIONS

- Use manipulatives, checklists, and charts. Have them easily accessible to supplement lesson plans or support individual academic activities.
- Post frequently used mnemonic devices in the classroom.

Impulse Control

Children who struggle with this subset of EFs often appear to be misbehaving (Dawson & Guare, 2010). They struggle to pay attention to work, are easily distracted, frequently get out of their seat, or blurt out answers or statements. It can be easy to assume these behaviors are the result of being willful or difficult, but these children are often frustrated with themselves. In order to support the development of successful coping strategies and a positive sense of self, the following steps can be employed.

1. Work with the student to identify the behavior and the trigger for the behavior.
2. Assess if any of the triggers can be removed. Develop awareness by working with the student to understand the connection between the trigger and their behavior.
3. Work together to make a list of replacement behaviors.
4. Practice the replacement behavior using role-play or simulations.
5. Encourage the student to use the new strategies/behaviors in low-stress environments.
6. Slowly encourage the student to use the new strategies/behaviors in increasingly stressful or intense situations.
7. Connect the use of the whole procedure to a reward. Use small rewards and praise at each step and an agreed-upon big reward when the new strategy/behavior is utilized in more stressful situations or when the targeted behavior has been ameliorated.
8. Provide verbal praise and encouragement throughout the process. Be sure to be honest and do not accidentally encourage the targeted behavior.

Based on: Dawson & Guare (2010).

This series of steps can also be used with entire classroom groups that struggle with specific impulsive behaviors.

SOCIAL/EMOTIONAL

The intention of EFs tutoring/training/development is for the students to eventually be able to monitor and regulate their own behavior without being dependent on adults or other individuals to do so. Fantuzzo et al. (1987) identified 11 elements of self-management interventions that can be integrated into the classroom and individual work. Follow-up studies indicate that these 11 elements are successful, especially when *every* element is employed. Importantly, including the student in the development of any plan to alter behavior increases the level of motivation and the likelihood they will develop increasingly independent self-management skills (Briesch & Chafoules, 2009). The 11 elements are:

1. Selection of a target behavior.
2. Creation of an operational definition of the behavior. How do you understand and describe the behavior?
3. Identify primary reinforcers of the behavior. What is the student "getting" from the behavior (avoidance of a task, attention, emotional expression, etc.)? Choose a new reinforcement for the desirable behavior.
4. Set a new goal. What do you actually *want* to be doing instead?
5. In real time, point out the behavior that was agreed upon to be reduced. Do so with compassion as opposed to guilt or shame.
6. Observe the target behavior.
7. Record the occurrence/frequency of the behavior.
8. Evaluate whether the goal for the replacement behavior has been met.
9. Use secondary agreed-upon reinforcers for the new desirable behavior.
10. When goals are met, use a primary reinforcer.
11. Monitor occurrence of behavior over time using visuals (charts or graphs).

The importance of including the student in the development of these plans should not be overlooked. Including their input develops metacognitive skills, provides motivation, and has been shown to be more effective. Methods for getting individual students involved in this process can be creative and fun, nurturing reflection and self-acceptance. During the development of these interventions, it is important to work honestly with the individual, but also provide examples of scripts that promote positive self-talk rather than destructive thought patterns.

Games that Support Development of Impulse Control

Jenga; Distraction; Mindtrap; AnimaLogic; Snake Oil; Quiddler; No Stress Chess; Simon Says; Red Light/Green Light; Musical Chairs; Freeze Dance; Chutes and Ladders; Candyland; Snap; Slapjack; Perfection; Duck, Duck, Goose!; Mother May I?; What Time Is It, Mr. Fox?; Remote Control Impulse Control; and Stare Junior.

ACADEMIC

Various subgroups of EFs have been found to correlate with both math and reading disabilities. This includes difficulty with inhibition, working memory, naming speed, and behavioral regulation (Desote & De Weerdt, 2013). In order to support a student's EFs, the method of instruction is often altered and specific strategies to manage the EF difficulty are taught. The activities suggested here are not specific instructional curriculum changes, but suggestions on how to support a child who struggles with both EF difficulties and a learning disability.

Reading – One way in which EF impacts reading ability is in reading rate. Children with EF struggles may read more slowly than their peers, but with external cueing are able to read at a more fluent rate. Once the cueing is removed, they may return to their slower rate. Also, comprehension is often impacted by poor EF skills. Direct instruction of self-monitoring skills as they relate to reading and multidimensional strategy techniques has been shown to be effective (McCloskey et al., 2014). Teach specific self-monitoring strategies. Also, support the student on multiple comprehension levels within content areas. This can be done by previewing vocabulary in game-like ways (use crossword puzzles and word searches once the vocabulary word has been defined). Model think-aloud strategies when encountering confusing text or ask questions about the content after reading a passage. When reading aloud, intentionally make "mistakes" to see if the students can "catch" you and correct you.

Math – Difficulties with self-monitoring, impulse control, and inhibition impact various areas of math skills. The student may misread operation signs or struggle to transpose numbers from one place on a paper to another. These students require support in organization and explicit instruction on self-monitoring their math skills. Important instructional steps include: help determine what is required for the math activity, discuss goals and strategies, model the strategy using mnemonics to help the student remember the strategy, practice the math strategy, and provide opportunities for independent practice of the skill (McCloskey et al., 2014).

Thinking Skills

Recall that this subset of EFs includes concept generation, reasoning and problem-solving, shifting sets (cognitive flexibility), fluency, and attention. There is considerable overlap with both working memory and impulse control.

Executive functioning allows for the planning and implementation of complex tasks. This involves deploying attention, which requires the regulation of arousal and vigilance, selective attention, sustained attention and attention span, as well as inhibition and control of behavior. In doing so, one is able to monitor performance and correct errors while simultaneously maintaining awareness of task-relevant information in the presence of irrelevant information. These abilities are essential to virtually all areas of academic performance (Korkman et al., 1998). While there is considerable overlap between EF difficulties and the full criteria for ADHD, it is important to remain aware of the differences and develop treatment plans and interventions accordingly. A common treatment for ADHD is the prescription of stimulant medication. The use of stimulants has been the most widely studied and prescribed psychotropic medication for children in the United States (Biederman et al., 1991; Safer et al., 1996). In addition to medication, children with attentional difficulties benefit from multimodal treatment that includes academic accommodations, parent training, behavioral intervention, social skills training

(Palumbo & Diehl, 2007), art therapy (Safran, 2002), psychotherapy (Gilmore, 2002), and mindfulness (Riner & Tanase, 2014).

Another EF subdomain that significantly contributes to the Thinking Skills category is cognitive flexibility. This involves the ability to disengage attention from one stimulus or activity and shift to another thought or action in response to change in the environment or task demands (Canas et al., 2003). This ability to flexibly shift has been connected to fluid intelligence (abstract reasoning) (Jones & Day, 1996). Difficulty in this area can result in rigid behaviors which manifest in displaying narrow interests, poor attention-switching, difficulty assimilating to change or novelty, and engagement in repetitive behavioral patterns (Baron-Cohen, 2008; Hill, 2004). It has been demonstrated that the ability to successfully manage these processes supports the development of social cognition (Yoshida et al., 2010). This relationship may be due to the complex interplay between EFs and emotion. For example, Mocan et al. (2014) found that individual differences in internalizing symptoms (anxiety and depression) played a role in children's ability to flexibly shift between emotional judgments. Given the interplay between EFs, social cognition, behavioral regulation, and abstract reasoning, it is easy to imagine how difficulties in this domain can impact functioning.

SOCIAL/EMOTIONAL

The preponderance of research regarding attention and social abilities generally focuses on ameliorating symptoms of ADHD, autism (joint attention and theory of mind), and traumatic brain injuries. The intent of this manual is to focus on functional domains used for successful daily behavior without focusing on DSM diagnoses. However, given the wealth of literature that focuses solely on attention, the following discussion and proposed interventions draw on research from these three diagnostic categories.

Imagine this scenario: a group of children play with various dress-up clothes and decide to write a play. They independently determine the setting and what sort of characters they will be and select tasks to complete. As they separate into their tasks, the one child charged with preparing the set is easily distracted, confused, loses track of the goal, and struggles to use materials from the environment (chairs, stools, blankets, toys, stuffed animals, etc.). After interrupting their friends several times with ideas for what *they* are doing or to ask questions about making the set, the child has managed to create a pile of seemingly random items on the floor and proudly presents their "set" to the group of children. They all blink, confused and unsure of how to respond.

This example demonstrates how a child's difficulty with thinking skills can impact their participation in a common social situation. This scenario is somewhat discrete, compared to more dramatic examples of how EF relates to social development. For example, attention regulation in infants and toddlers does or does not relate to the development of joint attention (Posner & Rothbart, 2007) or how shifting set (along with working memory and inhibition) can contribute to the emergence and/or expression of theory of mind (Carlson et al., 2015). It has also been demonstrated in teens and adults that similar yet distinct neural substrates are utilized during tasks that involved EFs (specifically planning accuracy, shifting sets, and inhibition of perseverative responses) and social cognition (Taylor et al., 2013).

It has been demonstrated that play-based intervention with 18-month-old children promotes the development of pro-social skills by fostering communication, connectivity, and problem-solving, in both the short and long term (Bundy et al., 2014).

Regarding cognitive flexibility, imagine the same scenario in which children are developing a "play" together. As ideas are tossed around and characters and plot develop, one child becomes fixated on a specific idea to act out a scene from their favorite movie. The movie scene does not relate to the ideas of the other children and, as the child becomes more insistent on including it, the others continue in their brainstorming and attempt to integrate the movie idea. However, the child simply cannot imagine altering any aspect of the scene. Eventually their frustration becomes extreme, evidenced by yelling at all the other children and storming off.

Difficulty with cognitive flexibility can manifest in several behaviors that can be difficult to manage. The individual may appear to be oppositional, defiant, unwilling to compromise, unwilling to follow directions, adhering strictly to routines, self-isolating, struggling to integrate the ideas of other people into their play, controlling conversation topics, or conversing on one topic longer than appropriate. It is important to remember that often it is not their choice to be rigid; their rigidity is based in a neurological underpinning. Their difficulty with rigidity can often lead to feelings of anxiety, which can then lead to more rigidity and an attempt to control the external environment. As a result, it is important to approach these individuals with empathy and compassion. Attempt to remain calm and do not interpret their behavior as personally insulting. At the same time, these individuals must develop awareness around how their actions impact people around them and learn more pro-social skills to manage their cognitive rigidity and subsequent emotional status.

Games that Support Development of Thinking Skills

Apples to Apples; Set; Ingenious; collectively alter rules to well-known games; rummy and gin rummy; poker; mahjong; Go; chess; Rubik's Cube; Sudoku; Puerto Rico; Clue; Skip-Bo; Concentration; Go Fish; 20 Questions; Headbandz; Break the Safe; Pictionary; Scattergories; TriBond Junior; Blokus; Oodles of Doodles; Imaginiff Jr.; Taboo; American Girl 300 Wishes; Whoonu; and Sync Up.

ACADEMIC

Some general academic guidelines for individuals who struggle with this aspect of EF include:

- Make the steps of all tasks/assignments specific. Stating "Write a paragraph about . . . " might be too general for students with EF difficulties. Break the task into small, manageable chunks.
- Avoid open-ended tasks.
- When cueing students that a new activity will start, include the materials they will need for the activity. If possible, post a visual reminder of what will be needed.
- Set aside instructional time to make lists of materials or assignments as a whole group.

Based on: Dawson & Guare (2010).

Reading – Thinking skills impact reading in several ways. For example, difficulty initiating reading tasks, maintaining focus and zoning out, and the inability to maintain interest and effort for reading passages, are all ways in which EF skills impact reading. Also, children with EF struggles often demonstrate an irregular reading rate (which involves fluency). They often read more slowly than their peers, but with external cueing are able to read at a more fluent rate. Once the cueing is removed, they return to their slower rate. Establishing connections between prior knowledge and new knowledge is another reading ability impacted by thinking skills (McCloskey et al., 2014). The impact of cognitive flexibility on reading skills has been researched with varying results that indicate some involvement in meta-linguistic, phonological, and print awareness; rhyming skills; early word reading; cross-modal connections between spoken and written language; and the ability to process phonological and semantic information simultaneously (Cole et al., 2014).

Math – Thinking skills impact math in ways similar to how they impact reading (initiation, zoning out, maintaining effort, etc.), especially when the math operations require reading skills (word problems). In addition to the issues previously listed, students may also struggle to identify solutions to math problems, despite having previously demonstrated knowledge of math concepts and adequate quantification and reasoning abilities. Students may also reverse numbers or incorrectly sequence them, operational signs may be inappropriately substituted, steps to problems may be inadvertently skipped, and writing may be illegible or so poorly organized that the student cannot find their place or read their own work (McCloskey et al., 2014). Students benefit from learning self-correcting strategies similar to those discussed in the Impulse Control section of this chapter.

ENVIRONMENTAL CONSIDERATIONS

- Provide prompts, both visual and verbal, that support organizational skills such as checklists, calendars, clocks/timers, and to-do lists.
- In spaces such as desks and bedrooms, develop organizational strategies, such as using colored masking tape to create boundaries within a desk. Clearly label what materials go within each boundary.
- Tape a list of organization strategies, materials, or expected behaviors on the student's desk. With the student, develop a reward system for successful completion of behaviors.

Chapter 3 Appendix: Executive Functioning Interventions

WHOLE-GROUP INCENTIVE PLAN FOR QUICK/QUIET TRANSITIONS

Goal: Facilitate transition from recess/special/other activity into the classroom.

Materials: Timer, posted checklist of expected behaviors, designated space in classroom to post times, large jar, colorful marbles.

Directions: Explain to the whole class that you have a new challenge for them. If the class has had difficulty with transitions, clearly state problem behaviors in a non-blaming matter-of-fact tone. Explain that part of good student behavior is how they enter the classroom and get ready for the next activity. To do so, they can play a game. Show the class a checklist of expected behaviors (include visuals if it is helpful). For example:

- Enter the classroom quietly at a medium pace (make sure you have defined medium pace, which can be done with a Simon says-style movement game).
- Go to your desk.
- Look at the schedule.
- Look at the list of materials you will need.
- Quickly and quietly get out the materials.
- Sit down and put your finger on your nose (or some other non-verbal gesture such as hands on shoulders or giving yourself a hug) to show you are ready.

Tell the students you will be timing the whole class, starting from when the bell rings, and will stop when they are all seated with their fingers on their noses. If they can do it quietly in less than _____ minutes, they will earn a marble in the jar. If they can beat their previous timed record, they will earn a bonus marble. If they are polite, kind, and supportive to each other they could also earn a bonus marble. When the jar is full, they will earn a fun classroom activity. Choose an activity that is motivating for the characteristics of that particular group (extra recess, a dance party, free art time, etc.).

After they have earned their first fun activity, allow the class to brainstorm activity ideas and create a "menu" that you will choose from for future activities. Send home a notification to the parent(s) regarding the plan, stating problem behaviors and the goal. Ask for their support and encourage the parent(s) to discuss the plan with their child. When the fun activity is earned, send home another notice encouraging the parents to praise their child.

WHOLE-GROUP END OF DAY ROUTINE

Goal: Facilitate organized transition at the end of the day to ensure students have homework assignments and all their materials.

Materials: Organizational notebook/binders, highlighters, checklist posted on board or on student desks.

Directions: Explicitly lead the students through each step. Pause after giving directions for each step, allowing for ample time. Praise the group with the successful completion of each step.

Step 1: Instruct students to retrieve their backpack and bring it to their desk.

Step 2: Direct students' attention to posted checklist or hand one out.

Step 3: Instruct students to open assignment book and compare their notes to what has been posted in the classroom.

Step 4: Direct students to fill in missing assignments.

Step 5: Direct students to highlight materials that are required for the assignment.

Step 6: Direct students to acquire each item, put it in their backpack, and check it off the list.

As the group and individual students get more secure with the routine, slowly fade out support. Encourage students to support each other. Ask the class, "What step comes next?" Prompt the class to begin the routine and check in with each child as they complete it.

Adaptations:

- Consider making the routine into a game or challenge. Time how long it takes for the whole group to complete the activity.
- Once familiar with the steps, invite a "student leader" to prompt the class.
- Sing the instructions, using a different "genre" of music each day (opera, rock, rap, etc.).

Based on: Dawson & Guare (2010).

INDIVIDUAL SELF-TALK DEVELOPMENT

Goal: Develop awareness of strengths and vulnerabilities, develop strategies for self-regulation.

Materials: Camera, printer, markers or pencils, Self-Talk Worksheet (see next page).

Directions: Explain to your student that you want to help them learn a new skill. State three clear ways in which their EF difficulties impact their daily life (forgetting things, handling frustration, perseverance). Give the student the choice of what they would like to deal with. Suggest a role-play in which they do the activity and you take pictures. Print out the pictures and together draw thought bubbles above their heads. Complete the Self-Talk Worksheet by drawing or writing. Help them to:

1. Name the problem.
2. State the plan.
3. Follow the plan.
4. Ask "How did I do?"

Once the worksheet is completed, take a phrase from the worksheet and write it in the thought bubble in the printed-out picture. Provide positive reinforcement during the activity and encourage the student to use the language in the moment during the school day.

Adaptations:

- Choose language that is meaningful and relevant to the individual. If possible, make it amusing to both of you.
- Develop a non-verbal cue that can be used to signal the student in real time to use the script you have developed.

Self-Talk Worksheet

Name: ______________________

1. What am I working on?

2. What is the plan? What can I say to myself that will help?

3. Am I following the plan?

4. Did I do the plan?

WORKING MEMORY: SOCIAL SKILLS GROUP INTRODUCTION

Goal: Facilitate learning names in a small group and develop working memory skills.

Materials: None. To be completed during a small group activity.

Directions: Ask the group to stand in a circle. Explain that this game will help everyone learn each other's names and communicate how they are feeling that day. Going around the circle, each person will say their name. After they have said their name, they will do a movement/gesture that describes their mood (do a few examples if this is confusing to the group). The whole group will repeat the name and gesture. Explain that once you have said your name, it will be your neighbor's turn, but you will build on the names and movements. The neighbor will say their name and movement, and then the whole group will say the leader's name/do the movement, and then copy their neighbor. Every group member will take a turn and the list of names/movements/gestures will grow longer and longer.

Adaptations:

- Rather than a movement or gesture, give the students small drums, chimes, etc., and they can tap out a rhythm.
- Add other props that facilitate the gesture (such as scarves).

WORKING MEMORY: READING COMPREHENSION – DRAWING

Goal: Promote understanding and recall of reading material.

Materials: Short story at the developmental level/grade level of the students, paper, and the students' preferred drawing medium.

Directions: Prior to reading the selection out loud to the class, preview any new vocabulary words with the classroom group. Provide definitions of the new words, both written and pictorial.

Introduce the story or text you are going to read to the class. Provide drawing materials. Instruct the students to draw a picture of the story as you read it. After you have finished reading the story, they will be encouraged to show peers their drawing and explain what they drew.

Adaptations:

- Ask the students to draw *after* the text has been read aloud. Before starting the drawing process, ask the children to imagine what they heard. Have them close their eyes and consciously picture images from the text. Once they have visualized the image, have them draw it. Ask them to explain what they drew.
- Provide more visual structure for the students using the graphic organizer on the following page.

Based on: Cain (2006).

Reading Comprehension: Drawing Worksheet

Name: ______________

First

Middle

Last

WORKING MEMORY: MATH FACTS

Goal: Promote automatic recall of math facts.

Materials: If possible, learn what sort of small toys, animals, or art materials the student is interested in. Have at least 20 of the items on hand. Large math flashcards.

Directions: Announce to the child/class that you are going to practice remembering math facts. Say, "We are going to practice remembering some math facts that you have already seen. We are going to practice how fast you can remember them in your head. This is not a race between each other, but a chance to practice for yourselves. I am going to hold up a math card and read the math problem aloud. For example, 3 + 7. In your head, try to picture three of your favorite toys [animals, food, etc.]. Then try to picture seven of your favorite toys. Once you do that, try to count them all to find the answer. Try it in your head first. If it is hard to do, use the toys that are on your desk. Once we are done practicing math facts, you will have some time to play with the toys." Go through all the math flashcards until the class fatigues and needs to take a break.

Based on: Alloway & Passolunghi (2011).

IMPULSE CONTROL: DEVELOPMENT OF AWARENESS OF TIME – INDIVIDUAL INTERVENTION

Goal: Facilitate the developing awareness of time and how long a task can/should take and encourage task initiation.

Material: Analog clock with Plexiglas face, dry erase markers of various colors.

Directions: Give the child a task that needs to be completed (cleaning a room, working on homework, completing a project). Estimate how long the task could take based on prior experience with the individual. Tell the child, "I need you to help me finish __________. I think it will take ________ [amount of time]. Let's draw on the clock how much time that will look like. Let's make the first ________ minutes green [or their preferred color] and the last five minutes, the 'warning, time is almost up' minutes, blue [or their preferred color]. When the task is all done or when the time is up, we can stop." After the first demonstration, allow the individual to draw on the clock.

Adaptations:

- Use the clock to indicate when breaks are taken.
- Provide an immediate reward upon completion of the activity. The award could be time spent together in a preferred activity, a small treat, or a small prize. This could be used as part of a larger behavioral plan, such as earning marbles. Once the jar is filled with marbles, a larger prize/activity could be earned.

Based on: Sarah Ward and Cognitive Connections, http://efpractice.com.

IMPULSE CONTROL: DEVELOPMENT OF AWARENESS OF TIME – GROUP INTERVENTION

Goal: Establish within a group setting expectation for task initiation and focus.

Materials: Analog clock with Plexiglas face, dry erase markers of various colors.

Directions: Indicate to the class that a task or activity will be starting soon (quiet work at their desks, stunted presentations, play time, etc.). Draw on the face of the clock the amount of time they will have to work on the task before switching to a new task or activity. Make the last five minutes of the task a different color. State the expectation that all students will stay on task and focus for the specified duration. Encourage the students to encourage and support each other.

Adaptations:

- Assign a student to the task of drawing on the clock for the week or day.
- Develop the expectation that the entire group will stay on task. Develop a reward plan for the entire class when they meet the expectation (earn marbles in a jar for a class party or extra recess).

Based on: Sarah Ward and Cognitive Connections, http://efpractice.com.

IMPULSE CONTROL: DEVELOPING AWARENESS OF EMOTIONAL/BEHAVIORAL RESPONSE TO A TRIGGER

Goal: Help identify triggers and emotional reactions to internal or external events.

Material: Thermometer Worksheet/manipulative.

Directions: With an individual, engage in a conversation about times they have had behavioral reactions that were inappropriate or difficult to manage. Try not to shame or blame the individual, but approach the conversation with empathy and compassion. Suggest that the feelings they have that lead to the behavior are valid, but that the intensity of the feelings leads to acting "out of control," and explain that you would like to help them "boss the feeling" so that it can stay in their control. During the conversation, help them:

- Identify the emotion and behavior (anger, anxiety, sadness, frustration, boredom, excitement, etc.).
- Identify the trigger for the feeling (sitting for a long time, behavior of peers, frustration with specific type of academic work or subject).
- Show them the Thermometer Worksheet or manipulative. Work with the individual to identify when the emotion is getting so "hot," "intense," or "big" that they can no longer control their behavior.
- Develop a plan of action to help prevent the emotion from hitting the "boiling point" or getting too big.
- Work with the individual to determine where the thermometer can be posted or placed in the room so it can be utilized in the moment.

Adaptations:

- Make sure the child is able to label their emotional experience. Before they can begin to identify triggers, they may need support in learning to recognize and label their emotions.
- Make the thermometer with the individual so they can personalize it or decorate it. Make the thermometer three-dimensional, using cardboard tubes and other materials.
- Role-play the plan that is developed to help manage the emotion.

Feelings Thermometer

Name: ________________

The emotion/feeling that is getting out of control is: ______________

The trigger for the feeling getting so big is: ______________________

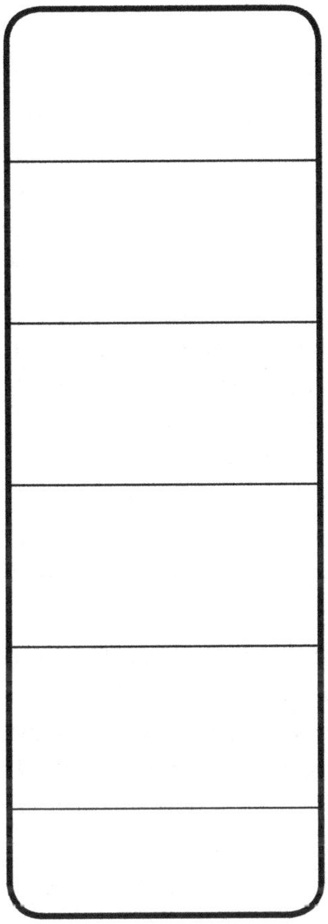

The feeling is too big to control! Help!

The feeling is starting to feel like it is too much.

I can feel the feeling but it is still okay. I can still focus on my work.

I can feel the feeling but it is pretty small.

I can hardly feel the feeling.

IMPULSE CONTROL: READING COMPREHENSION – TEACHING SELF-MONITORING SKILLS

Goal: Model and foster self-monitoring skills during reading comprehension.

Word Detective – While reading aloud, pause on an unfamiliar word. Write the word on the board and talk through the process of determining the meaning. Look for context clues, prefixes and suffixes, and the origin of the word. Confirm the definition of the word with a dictionary. This can be done in a game-like manner. Develop a name for the "game" with the group as part of the think-aloud strategy. Encourage the students to do the same thing when they get "stuck" in not knowing a word. Encourage them to involve the teacher or peers in the process.

Confusing Passages – Find a passage that is related to a current curriculum topic. Embedded within the excerpt, locate a confusing passage. While reading it aloud, pause and question the meaning of the passage. If possible, make sure the students have a copy of the passage, or display it on the board. Highlight the passage. While talking aloud, model strategies for making sense of it. Re-read the passage, pausing on clues. Study corresponding diagrams or pictures and relate the information to books you have read previously. This can be turned into a game.

Playfully write passages about the day or your students. Make sure certain passages or sentences are slightly confusing. Have the students edit your work and correct the comprehension mistakes. When the reading material is relevant or about students' own lives, motivation increases and allows them to feel held within the relationship.

Pause to Stop and Recall – Share with the class that sometimes while reading, you get to the end of the passage/page and realize you can't remember anything you've read. Ask them if they have ever done the same thing. While reading aloud, ask them to remind you to stop and remember what you've read. Encourage the students to read silently to themselves. Set a timer and when it goes off, have the students check in with each other and remember what they have read. This can be done in a game-like and fun style.

Question Brainstorm – After reading a passage or book, brainstorm with the group questions that developed as a response to the reading. Some can be silly and some can be informative or factual. In a narrative, question the behaviors, reactions, and motivation of the characters. Brainstorm ways that the answers to the questions can be found.

Attempt to keep the conversations short but meaningful. Identify the skill as self-monitoring.

Based on: Robb (2010).

DEVELOPING SELF-MONITORING SKILLS: MATHEMATICS

Goal: Promote self-monitoring skills as they relate to specific mathematic operations. Develop a checklist to ensure success and promote motivation.

Materials: Personalized checklist developed by the teacher or with the student(s), worksheet or assignment for current math curriculum.

Description:

Step 1. The teacher develops an understanding for how a student is completing specific math activities (worksheets, computation, word problems, etc.) and is/is not successful. Through observation, correction of work, interview, and asking the student to solve a problem using a "think aloud" method, the teacher can identify common errors made by the student. Based on this information, the teacher develops a four- or five-item checklist that addresses commonly made errors.

Step 2. Introduce the checklist to the student and integrate feedback. Work together with the student to practice using the checklist until they are able to use it independently. Allow the student to decorate or laminate the checklist. Provide positive feedback for using it. When assignments are completed, the student submits both the checklist and the work to the teacher.

Step 3. Provide praise for using the checklist and quickly give feedback on the quality of the work.

Step 4. (optional). If the student requires an incentive plan for utilizing the checklist, develop the plan with the student in the context of the relationship.

Step 5. If possible, fade the intervention once the student has reached the target performance level on the math operation.

Based on: Dunlap & Dunlap (1989), and Uberti et al. (2004).

THINKING SKILLS: SOCIAL/EMOTIONAL – THINKING BEFORE ACTING

Goal: Develop skills in decision-making and self-control. Teach the importance of thinking in advance and understand the connection between behavior and natural consequences (how others respond, lost or broken items, etc.).

Materials: Thinking Before Acting Worksheet, a book about self-control that is developmentally appropriate (some examples include: *My Mouth Is a Volcano!* by Julia Cook, *No, David!* by David Shannon and *The Girl and the Bicycle* by Mark Pett, which is an example of successfully thinking ahead). Chapter books can be appropriate as well.

Directions: Read a story that includes a character who behaves without stopping to think about their actions. Following the story, ask the group why it is important to think before acting. Brainstorm on the board. After the session, read a story about a child who made a plan to achieve a goal. Following the story, ask the group how the character made the plan and why it worked. Facilitate a discussion on thinking before acting and self-control. After the discussion, ask the children to complete the Thinking Before Acting Worksheet as a group or independently.

Adaptation: This activity can be broken into shorter time frames for children who have short attention spans or need movement breaks.

Based on: Shapiro (2004).

Thinking Before Acting

Name: ______________

Read the story and answer the question.

George was at school and about to eat the lunch he packed. When he opened his lunch box, there wasn't anything inside. George got mad and thought, "Who took my lunch?!?! I bet it was my brother! I'm gonna get him!" George surprised his friends when he stood up from the table, went to the other side of the lunch room where his brother was eating lunch, and started to yell at him.

How does George know his brother took his lunch? ________________

____

Does it sound like George is blaming his brother? ________________

____

Are there other possible explanations for where George's lunch has gone? What are they?

____

____

A group of kids were playing basketball during recess. Anna really liked basketball and really liked to win. While dribbling the ball, her friend Juan bumped into her and she fell, losing the ball. Anna got mad and yelled, "Foul! You did that on purpose!" She ran at Juan and pushed him down. "No, I didn't!" Juan said. "I tripped on my shoe lace!"

Why did Anna think Juan pushed her on purpose? ________________

____

What feelings might Juan have?________________________________

What could Anna have done differently after she fell? ______________

____

THINKING SKILLS: SOCIAL/EMOTIONAL – SELF-REFLECTION

Goal: Develop self-awareness and problem-solving strategies related to difficulties with EFs.

Materials: Artist-quality drawing paper and materials. This activity should take place over the course of several weeks. It can be helpful to provide a list of feelings.

Directions: In a small group or with an individual, let the student(s) know you are going to make a collection of drawings (it can also be referred to as a portfolio). This collection will be about things that are hard for them, things they like to do, and ideas on how things can feel better. One at a time, present the individual with a series of questions and ask them to draw their response. Questions can include: How does it feel to be bored? How does it feel to have a hard time paying attention to things? What does it feel like when you do something you're good at? How do you feel when other people seem to be frustrated with you? How does it feel when you say or do things you wish you could take back? What are some things you like about yourself? After each drawing, be sure to have a conversation with the individual about it and what it was like to make it. Do not make assumptions about the artwork without having a discussion with the individual.

Based on: Safran (2002).

THINKING SKILLS: PROBLEM-SOLVING – ADDRESSING COGNITIVE RIGIDITY

Goal: Facilitate social skill development around problem-solving. Reinforce that there can be multiple solutions to the same problem.

Materials: Many Solutions worksheet.

Directions: Have a conversation with the students about how to work through conflict with peers; for example, when two students want to play together but cannot agree on what to play. You can say, "Sometimes it is a good idea to think of several ways to solve a problem with a friend. It might not always be perfect; sometimes you'll get your way, and sometimes you'll have to be flexible even though it is hard. If you work together to find as many solutions as possible that seem good, you can try to use one that seems best. If it doesn't work, you already have another solution!" As a group, complete the following worksheet on finding multiple solutions.

Adaptation: Make worksheets that reflect the current interests and attitude of the group you are working with. Put in some social situations they have already overcome and some situations you could imagine happening. Also include some funny situations.

This language could be altered to include the word "compromise." Have a conversation about how, in a compromise, no one gets exactly what they want but that they both get a little of what they want. They have to meet in the middle. The idea of meeting in the middle could be acted out or displayed through an art project.

Many Solutions

Name: ______________

How many solutions can you think of?

Joy and Ricky want to play together but Joy wants to play a board game and Ricky wants to play with Legos.

Solution 1

Solution 2

Solution 3

Marcus and Greg both want to sit at the same desk or chair. Who gets it?

Solution 1

Solution 2

Solution 3

THINKING SKILLS: MANAGING RIGID BEHAVIOR AND COGNITIVE INFLEXIBILITY

Goal: Increase cognitive flexibility and de-escalate rigid behaviors.

- Set clear expectations prior to academic or social activities.
- Develop language with the individual that addresses the cognitive rigidity, helping them develop awareness around how their thinking and behavior impacts the people around them. Do this with compassion and lack of judgment.
- Helpful language could include, "Sometimes when you are doing your work or playing with friends, you get stuck on your own ideas. When you get stuck, you don't look happy. We want to help you learn how to get unstuck so you can be with people in a way that feels good to you and everyone around you. This takes practice! We can help you practice."
- With the individual, develop clear behavior plans that address specific issues of observed rigidity.
- Be consistent and follow through.
- Avoid direct confrontation or arguing. Use humor, redirection, and creative problem-solving to de-escalate potential behavioral issues.
- Praise all instances of cognitive flexibility.
- Planned ignorance.
- Try to identify underlying emotional triggers for instances of rigging (anxiety, frustration, confusion, excitement, etc.). Help the child identify the triggers and develop more pro-social responses.

THINKING SKILLS: CLASSROOM INTERVENTIONS - DEVELOPING INTENTIONAL THOUGHT

Goal: Through the use of frequent, short-duration, and informal meditative practices, foster self-discipline and control over the thought process. The following exercises are intended to encourage the ability to maintain focus, "bring the mind back" to a task, develop awareness, and provide opportunities throughout the school day to refocus.

- When the class has lost focus, have the students take a series of deep breaths. Teach them "balloon breathing," quiet and deep slow breaths in which they breath in and out completely. While in front of the group, use your hands to mime blowing up a balloon and the controlled release of air. Do four or five breaths.
- When beginning an activity that is difficult or unpleasant (or one that is very pleasant), explicitly ask the students about their thoughts ahead of time. Develop imaginary labels for the thoughts. Discuss how these types of thoughts might be "normal," but are they helpful? Challenge the students to develop substitute thoughts that will help complete the work.
- Instruct students to close their eyes and "make a wave of cold water [or warm stones or tingles]" move from their toes to their heads. Then make the feeling move from one arm (or one set of fingertips) to the other. Then from their toes to their ears.
- Have the students drink water but challenge them to drink it in exactly 30 "same size" sips.
- Instruct the group to close their eyes and imagine themselves (or someone else) being happy. "What are you [they] doing? Why are you [they] happy?"
- Ask the students to stand on their tip-toes for as long as they can while they sing (or hum) their favorite song.
- "Breathe just loud enough that neighbors can hear the breathing. As you breathe in, imagine the air as one color and the exhaled air as another color."
- Have the students suck on a piece of candy. "Do not bite it; let it dissolve naturally. See how long the candy takes to dissolve when you do not 'eat' it." Time the length and develop charts to see if the time is always the same or if it varies. Instruct the students to note the flavor: does it taste the same when eaten quickly versus slowly? Does it taste the same if a new thought or idea pops into their head?

Based on: Riner & Tanase (2014).

THINKING SKILLS: READING RATE ACTIVITIES

Goal: Increase reading automaticity and develop fluency skills.

Activity 1: Timed Repeated Reading – Using a short passage of a text, have the student read the text multiple times while being timed with a stopwatch. Choose text that is at or just below the student's reading level and that also matches the student's interests and maturity level. Avoid using poetry for this activity because it is often read at different rates. Chart the rate at which they read each time to display improvement. Make the activity game-like. Invite the student to make the chart with you and decorate it to their preferences. This activity can be done one-to-one with an adult or with peers timing each other. If having students read in pairs, give each student different reading passages to avoid direct competition. For beginning readers, engage in untimed repeated reading.

Activity 2: Tape-Assisted Reading – Choose an audiobook that is slightly above the student's reading level and which is read at about 80–100 words per minute. Allow the student to read along as they listen. If possible, avoid using audiobooks that have music and background noise. Once the student is familiar with the text, have them read the book aloud along with the audiobook. Once they are able to read at the same rate as the audiobook, record them reading the book to provide feedback. This activity can work well with content-area books, exposing the student to content vocabulary words and repeated exposure to curriculum content.

Activity 3: Partner Reading – Have different students read aloud to each other. Pair stronger readers with those who struggle with fluency. Using a text that is at a slightly lower instructional level, have the stronger reader read first then have the less-fluent reader read the same passage. In another version of partner reading, two students are paired together and instructed to re-read a book or passage that the teacher has already read to the class. They can alternate pages or paragraphs. This type of activity can be done as part of a literacy block or using content-area material during science or social studies.

Based on: "Reading First in Professional Development," www.readingfirst.virginia.edu/prof_dev/fluency/section2.html.

–4–

Memory Interventions

Introduction

Memory is a process that "involves the complex of systems by means of which an organism registers, stores, retains, and retrieves some previous exposure to an event or experience" (Lezak, 1995, p. 429). Studies over the last several decades have identified memory as consisting of a number of dimensions with specific neuroanatomical correlates (Squire, 2004). As described in a previous publication (Reinstein & Burau, 2014), at least three types of memory are understood to be operative in our daily lives.

Explicit or Declarative Memory involves the conscious recall of a life event or learned knowledge (Squire, 1982). This is the kind of memory that allows us to recall our home address or phone number.

Implicit or Procedural Memory is the unconscious or unintentional recall of verbal, non-verbal, or visual motor sequences such as use of a native language, riding a bike, or playing a sport (Roediger, 1990).

Emotional Memory employs additional neural circuitry and can impact both explicit and implicit memory by heightening the salience of an event and facilitating storage, retention, and retrieval (Barrett & Bar, 2009).

These types of memory are distinct but interrelated. Research supports the idea that both explicit and implicit memory systems are present and functional from early infancy and develop in concert (Rovee-Collier, 1999), but may reach functional maturity at different ages (Lum et al., 2010). A system comprised of the amygdala and other subcortical structures appears to mediate the development of emotional memory, develops in early infancy, and is refined over the course of a child's development (Carver, 2013). While these distinctions in memory systems are significant from a theoretical perspective, it is important to note that each can be understood within the context of both short- and long-term memory development.

For the purposes of this manual, and consistent with our intention to provide a pragmatic approach to intervention based on observation and evaluation results, rather than chart a developmental course for the three memory systems defined above, it is more useful to delineate between the developmental course of short- and long-term memory and explore how these memory systems impact the learning process. This is how memory assessments most often approach this functional domain.

While the definition of **Short-Term Memory** or **Immediate Memory** overlaps with that of working memory, for our current purposes, we will define the former as creating memory representations rapidly, storing a limited number of representations at one time and requiring active rehearsal to maintain representations beyond a few seconds (Ross-Sheehy et al., 2003; Oakes & Luck, 2014). A discussion of working memory and its developmental sequelae were presented in the previous chapter.

Long-Term Memory or **Delayed Memory** can be understood as the ability to encode, consolidate, store, and retrieve information (Lukowski & Bauer, 2013). It includes an extensive reservoir of knowledge and a record of past experiences (Cowan, 2008). Memory representations are formed slowly, storage capacity is essentially unlimited, and memories suffer from little or no decay of information (Ross-Sheehy et al., 2003).

Observing Memory Skills

The following list of questions can be asked while making daily observations to help identify an individual's strengths and vulnerabilities.

Short-Term Memory

Observations that may indicate difficulty with short-term memory are often similar to those of working memory. To determine if the issue is related to working memory or short-term memory, remember that working memory requires the individual to *work* on the information, while short-term memory does not. For a list of questions relevant for short-term memory, refer to Chapter 3 and the section on working memory observations.

Long-Term Memory

- Are they slow to remember names of people, objects, or events?
- Do they struggle to memorize or retain new facts?
- Do they have difficulty remembering step-by-step procedures?
- Do they struggle to remember details?
- Do they struggle to recall information during tests?
- Do they struggle to remember nursery rhymes or stories?
- Do they struggle to rapidly name well-known objects?
- Do they require prompts or cues to recall what they know?
- Do they struggle to remember the sequence of events?
- Do they struggle to remember information presented in class?

Based on: Dehn (2012).

Observation and Development of Memory

When considering the development of memory skills, it is important to understand that a significant number of additional factors, such as organizational ability, ability to rehearse information, and elaboration skills, play crucial roles in performance and that development of these skills influences changes in performance with age (Schneider & Pressley, 1997; Schneider & Ornstein, 2015). Research over the last several decades has also revealed that memory skills develop much younger than previously thought (Rovee-Collier, 1999). Although it is very difficult to distinguish between various forms of memory at early ages, "a high-functioning memory system is in place before language is available for encoding and reporting information" (Schneider & Ornstein, 2015, p. 192). Children's ability to recall past experiences in conversation develops rapidly between the ages of 2 and 4 (Schneider & Ornstein, 2015).

Because the research on early memory development does not reliably distinguish between short- and long-term memory as well as between declarative, procedural, and emotional memory, Table 4.1 does not address these memory types in the early years. The distinction between visual and verbal short- and long-term memory becomes more relevant and better measured as children enter school-age years and, therefore, the chart will reflect that information. Furthermore, when considering these subdomains in respect to testing instruments, measures of short-term or immediate memory are made using tests that require recall of information immediately after presentation; for example, repeating a sequence of numbers or drawing a design before any interfering task is presented (short-term memory span). Long-term or delayed memory requires that the evaluee recall information presented 20 to 30 minutes or up to 24 hours previously, depending on the particular testing instrument. Lastly, the developmental chart below will focus on short- and long-term verbal and visual memories that are measurements of conscious or declarative memory, also known as event memory, which is the process associated with learning within an educational context. For a more detailed description of individual subtests that target specific aspects of verbal and visual memory, please refer to Reinstein and Burau (2014).

TABLE 4.1 Memory Development

Age	*Long-Term Verbal Memory*	*Long-Term Visual Memory*	*Short-Term Verbal Memory*	*Short-Term Visual Memory*	*Assessments*
5–8 years	• Children have better narrative recall for logically, rather than randomly, connected events • Prior knowledge of an event increases storage and recall of a new event • Highly elaborative reminiscing of an event between mother and child results in children with richer memories about personal experiences	• In second grade, a student's visual unit for word recognition is a component letter-by-letter recognition rather than the whole word	• Short-term memory span of four items (digits, letters, words) • Ability to recall about 15 sentences on a sentence span test	• Rapid improvement in ability to recall or recognize previously seen visual patterns • Slower improvement in recall of visual information when required to remember where it was located in space (visual spatial patterns) • Ability to recall two pattern locations on a visual association test	• California Verbal Learning Test (CVLT) • Children's Memory Scale (CMS) • Wide Range Assessment of Memory and Learning (WRAML) • Test of Memory and Learning (TOMAL) • A Developmental NEuroPSYchological Assessment-II (NEPSY-II) • WJ-IV-COG • WISC-V • SB-5 • KABC-II

(continued)

TABLE 4.1 *(continued)*

Age	*Long-Term Verbal Memory*	*Long-Term Visual Memory*	*Short-Term Verbal Memory*	*Short-Term Visual Memory*	*Assessments*
9–12 years	• With age, children focus more on novel aspects of events and less on routine aspects • Forgetting of early childhood experiences has peaked and begins to stabilize	• In sixth grade, a student's visual unit of word recognition is the whole word	• Short-term memory span of six items • Ability to recall about 25 sentences on a sentence span test	• More rapid improvement in recall of visual patterns and slower improvement of visual spatial patterns • Ability to recall four pattern locations on visual association test	• CVLT • CMS • WRAML • TOMAL • NEPSY-II • WJ-IV-COG • WISC-V • SB-5 • KABC-II
12–18 years	• Developing cognitive and social skills enables the development of a life narrative that includes ability to take perspective and integrate emotions		• Short-term memory span increases to adult level of seven items • Ability to recall about 35 sentences on a sentence span test (adult level)	• Recall of up to five and a half items on a block sequencing task • More rapid improvement in recall of visual patterns and slower improvement of visual spatial patterns continues	• CVLT • CMS • WRAML • TOMAL • NEPSY-II • WJ-IV-COG • WISC-V • SB-5 • KABC-II

Sources: Schneider (2015), & Samuels & Eisenberg (1981).

Developing Accommodations and Interventions

Once a child's strengths and vulnerabilities in memory have been identified through observation and assessment, accommodations can be put in place and interventions can be made. The following sections indicate specific interventions. Always individualize the accommodations and interventions and remember the overlay of social/emotional functioning. Furthermore, it is important to remember that all of the following accommodations and strategies are best implemented within the context of a holding environment (Winnicott, 1965) that has a foundation based in the relationship formed between the teacher or specialist and the child.

General Academic Accommodations and Strategies

The following list of accommodations and strategies can be implemented in the classroom. Some of these accommodations can be included in an IEP or 504 plan.

- Break information into small manageable chunks.
- Allow use of a cheat sheet during tests.
- Allow use of calculator.
- Allow use of manipulatives.
- Allow open-book assessments or tests.
- Use cloze procedure with a word bank, matching, true/false (yes/no) and multiple-choice during assessments or tests.
- Provide a source of external memory (handwritten or typed notes, writing on the whiteboard or Smart Board).
- Allow access to formula sheets during tests.
- Provide a written or pictorial list of steps for a task.
- Check for comprehension after providing directions.
- Provide reminders for specific tasks (alarm on cell phone, rubber band around wrist, etc.).
- Use a daily planner.
- Provide a visual classroom schedule.
- Encourage the student to ask questions.
- Underline or highlight important information in text.
- Mark text with Post-It notes or flags.
- Provide lecture notes.
- Allow/provide recording device for lectures and labs.
- Allow extra time for tests/exams.
- Allow extra time for assignments when negotiated in advance.
- Reduce course load.
- Allow access to technology for mind-mapping software.
- Frequently drill and review material.

Short-Term Memory Accommodations

- Provide preferential seating away from distractions.
- Use simplified language while giving directions.
- Provide visual supports for directions.
- Write important information on the board.
- During lecture, provide a formatted and written script with blanks that the student can complete as the lecture is given.
- Provide multimodal instruction.

Short-Term Memory Reading Accommodations

- Provide a table of facts for expository text.

Short-Term Memory Writing Accommodations

- Use word banks.
- Use graphic organizers.

Long-Term Memory Accommodations

- Frequently review learned material.
- Utilize multiple instructional modalities (writing, listening, kinesthetic, integration of sensory experience).
- Allow extra time for rehearsal.
- Provide visual references.

Long-Term Memory Reading Accommodations

- Pre-read textbook material and preview vocabulary words.

Sources: Seaman (2014) and Dehn (2011).

Addressing Memory

In young children, memory difficulties often occur as secondary issues related to attention, verbal processing, visual perception, or general low global intelligence (Korkman et al., 1998). However, through the observation/assessment process, the student's preferred sensory process for taking in and encoding information can be revealed. In a classroom setting, this is most often through either visual or auditory modalities, as indicated in the developmental chart at the beginning of this chapter. People may also process information through the kinesthetic/tactile sensory systems. Understanding if a student's memory is most supported by visual, auditory, or kinesthetic/tactile stimuli is the first step to addressing issues related to memory and to utilizing the student's strengths. The ability to encode information is also related to a student's emotional state and level of motivation (Sprenger, 2005). The following section provides suggestions for utilizing the student's preferred sensory modality and developing a strong positive emotional connection to information.

General Interventions for Memory Skills

Supporting learning for students who struggle with memory (and those who don't) can be based on seven steps intended to support short-term memory and encode information into long-term memory stores (Sprenger, 2005).

1. Reach – Get the student's attention by introducing topics in a way that is meaningful, using their preferred sensory modality.
2. Reflect – Through the preferred sensory modality, provide opportunity for student to make connections between new information and prior learning.
3. Recode – Have student put the new information and ideas into their own words and expression.
4. Reinforce – Provide positive reinforcement; give both formal and informal feedback to avoid misconceptions.
5. Rehearse – To promote higher-level thinking and incorporation of multiple memory systems, engage student in related activities.
6. Review – Use games, practice tests, writing exercises, mind-mapping, roleplaying, and drawing to offer multimodal review opportunities.
7. Retrieve – Ask student to remember new information and apply it in different ways.

In addition to these strategies, it can be effective to specifically teach students about memory, how it works, and the difference between short- and long-term memory. This is referred to as "meta-memory" (Schneider, 2010). Meta-memory also includes self-awareness of one's own memory strengths and weaknesses, such as understanding that visual information may be preferred over auditory and vice versa. This also includes the awareness of the type of memory strategies that are most successful from individual to individual (Dehn, 2011). Increased meta-memory often corresponds with an increase in the use and application of memory strategies (Harris, 1996). For example, an individual who doesn't believe any and all memory strategies are effective is less likely to invest time in learning such strategies. It can be important to assess an individual's perspective (meta-memory) regarding memory. The individual's perception of meta-memory can impact their social/emotional functioning, which in turn can impact their academic functioning. A common misperception of many students is that poor memory skills are equivalent with being "stupid" (Posner & Rothbart, 2007). The lack of awareness that memory is part of a constellation of skills that leads to academic success can instigate an unhelpful cycle that threatens a student's self-image (Autin & Croizet, 2012). As a result, interventions must include instructional and environmental practices and also support the student's developing self.

General Environment Considerations for Memory

- Post daily, weekly, or monthly schedule using words, graphs, and images.
- Promote the development of daily habits (using procedural memory) but placing visual cues in the environment (such as images for the steps to brushing teeth or daily decluttering of a backpack).
- Take photographs of people, places, and events. Put the photographs in the environment. If appropriate, label them or put them in sequential order.
- If possible, preview trips to new places or activities using photographs.
- Use multi-sensory teaching and manipulatives whenever possible.
- Make the environment uncluttered and reduce overwhelming visuals.

Emotional and Social Impact of Short- and Long-Term Memory

Our memory impacts various areas of emotional and social life. It contributes to remembering people, places we have been, and things we have done. Recollection of conversations, another person's food preferences, or birthdays and outings is part of the relationship. Memory holds important aspects of our lives and contributes to how we think about ourselves and the people around us and how we interact with the environment.

Autobiographical memory is another component of memory that is often not directly assessed but which plays a significant role in daily functioning. This type of memory combines episodic memory (personal experience) and semantic memory (factual information) to create the life story of an individual (William et al., 2008). This type of memory impacts our daily functioning in a variety of ways. How many times have you started a conversation with, "How was your day?" In doing so, you're asking the individual to recall events, locations, and feelings about an experience and their impressions. Autobiographical memory plays a role in various psychological and neurological disorders including amnesia, traumatic brain injury, post-traumatic stress disorder (PTSD), and various types of neurocognitive disabilities.

While working with children who have had significant difficulty in school settings or who have experienced traumatic life events, it is important to be mindful of how these experiences have impacted their development. Often, autobiographical memory is disrupted as being less conceptually connected to the event(s), resulting in a disorganized sense of the experience (Ehlers & Clark, 2000). Consequently, these memories can lack spatial, temporal, and causal context and are less detailed and disintegrated. Memories related to traumatic events can be more connected to sensory, perceptual, and emotional impressions, which can be triggered by similar cues (both internally and externally) pulling forth an intrusive or involuntary quality (van der Kolk, 1994). These intrusive memories can be extremely disruptive to an individual's daily experience.

Therapeutically addressing traumatic memories can be a complex long-term process that is beyond the purview of this book. However, within an academic environment it is essential to be mindful of a student's life experiences and be aware of how traumatic memories might impact daily functioning and contribute to the development of meaningful relationships. This awareness is part of the holding environment that can facilitate relational growth and support maturation (Winnicott, 1965). Trauma research also indicates that the development of a safe relationship works to bring the brain back into a regulated state and promotes healthily neurobiological development (van der Kolk, 2014). There are several ways in which interacting with an individual who is managing traumatic memories can facilitate growth as well as develop a safe and secure environment.

Short-Term Memory Interventions

Games that Promote Short-Term Memory

Chess; jigsaw puzzles; matching card games (use both neat rows and also messier arrangements); Sudoku; Simon Says; Bop It; Concentration; physical exercise, especially games that require the individual to cross the mid-line; and picture-comparison games in which one image is presented followed by another in which items have been added, subtracted, or changed.

ACADEMIC

Reading – Children with reading issues often have a limited auditory memory span (Korkman et al., 1998). This impacts the development of phonemic awareness and the association between letters as symbols and corresponding sounds. Short-term memory struggles can interfere with the acquisition of letter- and word-identification skills. It can also hinder the comprehension of long reading passages (Flanagan et al., 2002).

To support reading fluency in students who struggle to develop the symbol/sound association, teach students to recognize sight word vocabulary. This leads to better reading and greater fluency than having to decode (sound out) each word. This fluency develops based on attention and working memory (Kilpatrick, 2014). Reading interventions should be tailored to support word recognition skills (Mascolo et al., 2014). Helping students develop these skills enhances fluency, which is thought to provide a bridge between the development of word recognition and comprehension (Raskinski, 2012).

Math – Difficulties with short-term memory can impact math performance in various ways. In general, this functional domain contributes to the recall of mathematical procedures and facts. It has been specifically demonstrated that difficulties in visual short-term memory and working memory predict math achievement (Riccio et al., 2010). Auditory/verbal short-term memory plays a significant role when a student attempts to remember a sequence of orally presented steps of long math problems (i.e., first multiply, then add, then subtract . . .) (Flanagan et al., 2002). You can support multi-step directions by using both verbal and visual strategies (cue sheets, example problems, and posted steps for problems in the current math unit). The use of repetition and rehearsal has been shown to enhance recall of facts (Dehn, 2011). For activities that are repetitious, it is important to keep the student engaged and motivated (Bryant et al., 2014).

Long-Term Memory Interventions

Games that Promote Long-Term Memory

Crossword puzzles; verbal games such as "I'm going on a picnic and I'm taking . . . "; Jeopardy; Trivial Pursuit; vocabulary review games; and Which Came First?

ACADEMIC

During instructional periods, be sure to activate prior knowledge to enhance understanding. This can be done by:

- Asking questions about the topic.
- Asking questions about personal experiences or relating yours.
- Holding brainstorming sessions to identify what the students already know.
- Asking students to make opinion statements about the topic.
- Reviewing information at the start of an instruction session.
- Reviewing learned material in a variety of multimodal ways. For example, reinforce learned material using a video, making art, or roleplaying.
- Employing mnemonic devices to help students retain information.

Reading – Long-term memory plays a role in quickly naming objects or categories of objects. Individuals who struggle with this automatic recall require support to develop strong reading skills. Associative memory (consistently connecting a letter shape to the associated sound) is another long-term memory skill that is important for reading (Flanagan et al., 2002).

Math – Long-term retrieval abilities are important for math calculation skills (Flanagan et al., 2002). This is the ability to remember and recall math facts, steps to procedures and various mathematical rules, and to recognize different functions. Strategies used to address long-term memory deficits in math are similar to those used to address short-term memory.

Chapter 4 Appendix: Memory Interventions

BUILDING META-MEMORY

Goal: Promote and enhance the understanding of memory functioning, help students identify strengths and vulnerabilities, and utilize memory strategies. Promote meta-memory development.

Materials: Tray or plate, 5 to 20 small items the students are familiar with, cloth or towel, paper and pencil, piggy bank or some sort of vault.

Directions: Arrange five items on a tray and cover them with a cloth or towel. Instruct the group, "Let's do an experiment with our brains! Don't worry, it's going to be safe. Under my cloth there are a couple of different items. I am going to move the cloth and I want you to look at the items and try to remember them. You'll have [time] to look at them. After the timer goes off I will cover them again. Then I want you to quietly and independently write down as many of the items as you can. When everyone is done, I'll reveal the items and you can see how many you remembered." Repeat the activity, adding items and viewing time, until the group begins to struggle with remembering. As you do the activity, repeat the instructions.

Following the activity, have a group discussion. Define this skill as short-term memory. Specify this as a visual version (it mostly uses your eyes) of short-term memory. To demonstrate auditory/verbal memory, read a short story (three or four sentences long) and ask students to recall facts after hearing it. Read longer and longer passages until the group begins to struggle. Define this as auditory/verbal (it mostly uses your ears) short-term memory.

Help the students make the connection between learning new things and using their visual and auditory/verbal memory. On a piece of paper, write down "Memory Experiment." Show the class the piggy bank/vault. Explain that "You use long-term memory when you want to remember information for a long time. With short-term memory, you don't have to. Long-term memory is like a bank. It helps you save important things. We don't need to remember every item on this tray [put items away from the bank/vault]. We do want to remember all of our names. Please write your name on a small piece of paper and put it in the bank/vault."

During other instruction periods, when you introduce mnemonic devices or while playing other memory games, remind students of this activity. Write information that should be encoded into long-term memory on pieces of paper and place them in the bank/vault.

Adaptations:

- The "read a story and remember facts" and "piggy bank/vault" part of the lesson could be done during a separate instruction period if the classroom group has a short attention span.
- Have the students make their own bank/vault. Use this to facilitate other mnemonic devices (such as visualization and method of loci found in the next activity).
- If the group is larger, instead of a tray with items on it, project images onto a screen. Images should be of familiar places and items. The first image is the control image and the second is missing items or items that have been changed.

Based on: Neuroscience for Kids: Memory Experiments. Retrieved from https://faculty.washington.edu/chudler/chmemory.html.

SUPPORTING INDIVIDUALS WITH TRAUMATIC MEMORIES

Goal: Establish an environment that is perceived as safe and supportive. Begin developing a safe and supportive relationship.

Relaxation Training – Provide opportunities throughout the day to educate and practice relaxing. Techniques such as deep breathing, progressive muscle relaxation, positive images, and mindfulness can help students with affect regulation. The feelings thermometer discussed in previous chapters can also be used to help students identify when they have been triggered and what strategy to employ to re-regulate themselves.

Teach Problem-Solving – Intrusive memories, physiological arousal, hypervigilance, and increased anger/irritability can contribute to impulsivity or aggression. Learning useful problem-solving strategies (in a non-blaming empathic way) can help students mediate social and educational difficulties.

Classroom Environment – Have a safe and consistent routine that is predictable. Try to establish structure and avoid deviations. Within the room, provide a safe and quiet space that is comfortable and separate from the other students/people. Provide tactile sensory toys as recommended by an occupational therapist. Find out what types of music, toys, activities, and stuffed animals the students find relaxing, and attempt to provide them.

During Interactions – Remain quiet and calm and avoid startling the student or yelling. Try to avoid complex language, especially when the student is triggered. Set clear expectations of your relationship, maintain boundaries and follow through. Attempt to avoid interpreting their aggressive/irritated behavior personally. Model calming strategies throughout the day. Give students opportunities to make choices and create an atmosphere of respect.

Based on: Kataoka et al. (2012).

LONG-TERM MEMORY: TYPES OF MNEMONIC DEVICES

Goal: Help the student develop strategies for encoding information into long-term memory.

Repetition – The student repeats/rehearses information (orally, writing, drawing, singing, etc.) several times. This is most beneficial if it happens shortly after the learning and occurs intermittently thereafter.

Acronym – The student/group makes a silly or familiar saying to help them remember facts, especially those that can appear as a list. Use the first letters of words to make a phrase. For example, the names of the planets (*My Very Elderly Mother Just Sat on Uncle Ned*) or the names of notes on a musical scale (*Every Good Boy Deserves Fudge*).

Method of Loci – Have the students imagine themselves in a location that is familiar to them. They then imagine placing an object, word, or element related to the lesson in a prominent location within the imagined environment. When it is time to recall the information, ask the students to mentally retrace their imaginary trip and picture where they placed the object, word, or element.

Acrostic – The students recall a list of words or terms by making an actual word from the first letter of the words within the list. For example, *HOMES* may help them recall the names of the Great Lakes.

Visualization – Similar to Method of Loci, this mnemonic device asks the students to take a concept/term/sequence of steps and develop an associated mental image. It can be useful to have the students draw their visual representation and imagine the drawing at a later time. Use different colors or highlighters while the students review class or lecture notes to emphasize important information that is likely to be presented later. Teach the students to visualize the colorful page when attempting to remember the information.

Chunking – This is a method for breaking large pieces of information into smaller and more manageable pieces. For example, the 10 digits of phone numbers are clustered together in order to make them easier to remember. In the United States, it's a 3-3-4 cluster (555-970-9415). If asked to memorize a poem, break the poem into smaller pieces. Teaching students to look at numbers and letters or steps to problems in chunks can be a way to help them consolidate information.

Semantic Clustering – When the students are presented with large pieces of information or lists of words, help them organize the information into smaller groups or categories. For example, organize states by region. This process allows the students to recognize and group information into categories that are meaningful to them. Once categorized, the students can rehearse the information. Then, when attempting to recall the information, prompt them to follow the same sequence that they rehearsed.

Rhymes and Songs – A rhyme that has similar terminal sounds at the end of each line can help cue students to remember facts and words. Likewise, song rhythms and melodies can help cue students to remember lyrics, which could include facts and concepts.

Dual Encoding – Teach the students to use both visual and verbal strategies for the same information. If they are trying to learn new vocabulary words, ask them to speak and visualize them. If they are learning visual spatial information, such as the Periodic Table, ask them to speak their thoughts out loud or to make a narrative about the image.

Build a Narrative – When trying to remember a list of items, history facts or steps to solve a problem, develop a story or narrative that includes all the items and facts. Visualization can be included.

LONG-TERM MEMORY: STUDY TIPS FOR RETENTION AND RECALL

Goal: Develop several strategies for higher-level learning in order to retain and recall information in long-term memory stores.

Distributed Effort – Spread out studying over a number of days rather than cramming. Review at least some of the information on a test or exam a little every day.

State- and Context-Related Memory – Try to study/work in an environment that is similar to the testing/exam environment. Also try to be in the same physical state (well-rested and fed, for example).

Avoid Multi-Tasking While Studying – Try to attend to just the study materials while studying, especially dense material. Multi-tasking does not impact recall, but it does impact encoding. Divided attention impacts the encoding process.

Self-Quiz Frequently – Ask questions frequently. Every time a memory is accessed, it is strengthened. Self-quizzing will help identify areas that need strengthening and make memories more readily available for recall.

Individuality – Each person's memory works slightly differently. Try combinations of various strategies until the best mix is found.

Based on: Tigner (1999).

TEACHING WORD RECOGNITION SKILLS/SIGHT WORDS

Goal: Increase fluency by teaching word recognition and site word skills. Site words tend to be high-frequency words recognizable without using the phonological decoding process. Reading fluency can be increased if it is tough to recognize high-frequency words automatically. Teaching content-specific vocabulary words this way can increase reading fluency for all content.

Directions: Introduce three to five words at a time. Repeat various activities/strategies until the words are easily recognizable. Once the words have been learned, review frequently.

Word Walls and Flash Cards – Place three to five sight words on the word wall. Use the following strategies to introduce the word and reinforce it with various activities.

- See and Say: Have the student say the word while underlining it with their finger.
- Spell Reading: The student says the word, then spells it, then says it again.
- Arm Tapping: The student says the word, then spells it while tapping their arm as they say each letter.
- Air Writing: The student says the word, then writes the word in the air in front of them.
- Table Writing: Using their finger, the student writes the letters on the table, first looking at the word then not looking at it.

Use Manipulatives – Once words have been introduced, have the student use large magnetic letters to form them. Have them trace the word in a sand tray. Use stamps, letter cookie cutters, and play dough to form the word.

Put the Words in Context – Read stories or short passages that contain the words. With support, ask the student to highlight the words using markers or highlighting tape. Once the story is familiar, ask the student to independently locate the sight words.

Reinforce Words with Games – Have the students write the same word twice on separate flash cards (to make a matching pair of cards). In pairs or small groups, instruct the students to play Concentration by putting the cards face down and locating matches.

- In a similar way, create a Go Fish deck of cards.
- Make word searches that include the sight words.
- Make a Bingo board using sight words.
- Sight Words Pathways: Place flash cards on the floor. Have the student jump onto the card and read the word aloud. When they get the word correct, they can advance to the next word. Make the pathway twist and turn and jump around obstacles or onto chairs.

Based on: Mascolo et al. (2014); and Margurussa (2012).

MATHEMATICS AND MOTIVATION FOR FLASH CARDS

Goal: Support/motivate students to stay engaged during flash card drills. These ideas are designed for use with math facts, but can apply to other content areas.

Timing – When drilling math facts, do it while the student is at a good arousal level, such as right after getting some exercise, eating, or waking up refreshed from a nap.

Duration – Keep flash card drill times short but frequent. Five minutes three to five times a week is shown to be most effective. Long drill sessions that are intermittent and only done once weekly are less effective and less motivating.

Routine – Once you know the timing that works for the student/child and have a sense of how long they can maintain attention, build it into the weekly routine (such as right before lunch or right after recess). Whatever the timing is, make it part of the daily schedule.

Keep It Simple – Make sure the content of the cards (addition facts, for example) is presented in a simple way. If you are working on base 10 facts, only present base 10 facts. If you are working on skip counting by 2s, only use those addition facts. Develop groups or "families" and discuss with the student which number "families" you are working on.

Visual Effect – For students who have good visual processing skills and memory, make the number sentence a different color from the answer. For example, on one side of the flash card have "5 + 2 =" in red and the answer, "7", on the opposite side of the card in green. Ask the student what their favorite colors are and use those colors. For students who do not have strong visual processing or memory, make the cards as visually simple as possible.

Handmade – Have the students make the flash cards and, if appropriate, allow the students to use simple decorations. If the students struggle with graphomotor skills, allow them to use number stickers. Customize the flash cards to their interests. Think about how to add other sensory components to the cards. Make the numbers rough using sand or glitter or apply scent to the cards.

Combine Flash Card with Physical Activity – If they have added 6 + 3 = 9, allow the child to do nine jumping jacks, run in place for nine seconds, or do nine toe-touches. Another option is to have the child standing and, with each correct answer, take a giant step to the finish line. At the finish line, they might have a small prize or mystery item related to the content they are studying.

Make a Game Out of It – Put the cards in a fabric bag and have them pull the card out of the bag. Decorate the bag with their interests.

Be Present and Positive – Make sure *you* are able to attend to the flash card drills, provide feedback, and be engaged. Learn how the child likes to be praised. Use verbal compliments, noises, chimes, or bells that indicate correct answers. Do they need a small reinforcement after every card (one Skittle or M&M per card, or a small sticker) or a small reinforcement after the exercise drill is over (a sticker chart that earns them a homework-free day, extra recess or art time, a classroom party, a listen to one of their favorite songs, or something geared toward their interests)? As they develop stronger skills and employ them during instructional periods, be sure to praise them in that time and make a connection between flash card drills and their success in math work.

–5–

Visual Motor Functioning Interventions

Introduction

Anthony began attending a faith-based private preschool at the age of 4. He did well there until he began having difficulty in first grade. His distress increased significantly in second grade. He began having difficulty completing his work in school, struggling with homework and frequently becoming upset and angry. Anthony's second-grade teacher began punishing him by keeping him in from recess to complete his work, and became very disparaging to him. Anthony was so disturbed by this treatment that his parents transferred him to public school. While he initially did better, the increased demands for written output resulted in Anthony becoming increasingly distressed and, by the spring of third grade, refusing to go to school. Despite his parents' best efforts, Anthony refused to get out of bed or would run away and hide, or his parents' demands would trigger a panic attack. The school, with the full cooperation of Anthony's parents, put a series of behavioral plans in place to get him to school, none of which were successful. The school labeled Anthony a behavior problem and, at one point, reported the parents to the Department of Children and Family Services. At the time of testing, Anthony had not attended school for a year.

Testing was undertaken to better understand Anthony's resistance and emotional distress as well as any underlying neurological issues. While very cooperative and related, when asked to complete any tasks using paper and pencil Anthony made negative comments. When drawing symbols, he noted, "I can never do arrows, you found my weakness" and "I'm a really bad drawer, so it's going to look ugly." When asked to write a narrative on the Test of Written Language, Anthony panicked and was unable to write a story based on the visual cue. Instead, with much support and reassurance, he wrote a few barely legible sentences about one of his interests that bordered on obsession. Testing further revealed that Anthony's High Average Verbal and Visual Spatial abilities (88th and 77th percentiles, respectively) contrasted sharply with his Extremely Low Processing Speed Index (1st percentile). Furthermore, his score on the test of Visual Motor Integration was at the 0.7th percentile and he had very significant difficulty modulating size, pace, and precision, negotiating angles, and planning and spatial organization, a profile consistent with a diagnosis of dysgraphia.

While there are a number of different dimensions to the development of visual motor functioning, for our purposes we will focus on those that most directly pertain to skills encountered in the preschool and school environments. For a more detailed and broader discussion of visual motor development and functioning, the reader is referred to Reinstein and Burau (2014).

Looking at those visuomotor abilities that are relevant to academic skill development, can be assessed in a neuropsychological evaluation, and are amenable to intervention brings focus to the development of graphomotor skills and processing speed.

Graphomotor skills can be thought of as a subcategory of fine motor skills and their maturation is essential for the development of handwriting. According to Feder and Majnemer (2007),

> Failure to attain handwriting competency during the school-age years often has far-reaching negative effects on both academic success and self-esteem. This complex occupational task has many underlying component skills that may interfere with handwriting performance. Fine motor control, bilateral and visual motor integration, motor planning, in-hand manipulation, proprioception, visual perception, sustained attention, and sensory awareness of the fingers are some of the component skills identified . . . Studies of handwriting remediation suggest that intervention is effective. There is evidence to indicate that handwriting difficulties do not resolve without intervention and affect between 10 and 30% of school-aged children.
>
> (p. 312)

Processing speed is a measure of cognitive efficiency and relates to the speed with which an individual can execute basic cognitive processes (Kail & Ferrer, 2007). Research using developmental data and longitudinal models based in methods employing typical neuropsychological assessment tools indicates that, between the ages of 5 and 18, processing speed follows a quadratic pattern of growth (Kail & Ferrer, 2007). That is, it increases significantly in early to mid-childhood, continues to increase less rapidly by early adolescence, and reaches a peak rate of change in late adolescence (Kail, 1991). This maturational pattern has been correlated with the maturation of white matter in the brain (Ferrer et al., 2013). Furthermore, processing speed maturation relates to the development of multiple academic skills. For example, Lobier et al. (2013)

demonstrated that visual processing speed mediated by visual attention span predicted reading speed. Processing speed also has been found to predict speeded naming, visual processing, and phonological awareness (McBride-Chang & Kail, 2002). Droit-Volet and Zelanti (2013) found that processing speed was the best predictor of individual differences in awareness of time. It is important to consider, however, that accurate indicators of processing speed development may be task-dependent and influenced by culture (Kail et al., 2013).

While vulnerability in either of these functional domains can make school functioning a challenge, as dramatically displayed in the vignette above, vulnerabilities in both of these areas can make the writing process and school extremely distressing. In Anthony's case, the increasing demands for written output that began in second grade, the lack of awareness of the underlying issues, and the punitive approach to addressing his problems that continued into his new school with an inappropriate behavioral plan resulted in a level of trauma that fueled his resistance to school and undermined his self-esteem.

Observing Visual Motor Functioning

The following list of questions can be asked while making observations to help identify an individual's strengths and vulnerabilities in this functional domain.

Graphomotor Skills

- During writing activities, do they attempt to avoid the work or procrastinate through a variety of behaviors; for example, ask to go to the bathroom, re-sharpen their pencil numerous times, or get something from their backpack?
- During writing activities, do they sit and stare?
- During writing activities, do they disturb other children or frequently "get in trouble?"
- Do they frequently retrace letters or exhibit false starts or hesitancies while writing?
- Do they report difficulty in remembering what letters look like?
- What type of pencil grip do they use? Tripod grip? Hooked grip? Cylindrical grip? Digital grip? How efficient is the grip they are using?
- How tight or loose is the grip on the pencil?
- How hard do they press on the paper? Too hard?
- How closely do they look at the paper and pencil while writing? Do they put their face low to the table/writing surface?
- Can they write neatly, but often do not?
- Do they complain that their hand hurts while writing?
- Are they able to write with multiple speeds when necessary or do they only have one pace at which they write?
- Do they struggle to incorporate standards of capitalization, punctuation, syntax, and grammar into their written work?
- Do they find it easier to write in print or in cursive?

- Can they write at a level of their own speech? Can they convey their ideas in writing or does it limit their expression? Does their written vocabulary match their spoken vocabulary?
- Are all of their written passages short even if the requirements of the assignment are unmet?
- Is there the appearance of many careless errors?
- Do they struggle to use lined paper appropriately?
- Is there uneven spacing between letters or no spacing between words?
- Are there frequently misspelled words?
- Do they struggle to generate ideas during writing projects or elaborate upon their ideas?
- Do they struggle to understand the perspective of the audience?
- Do they struggle with writing tasks that require creativity and/or critical thinking?

Processing Speed

- Do they take longer to complete assignments than expected?
- Do they struggle to follow multiple-step directions?
- Are they unable to finish tests in the allotted time?
- Is it difficult for them to read and take notes simultaneously?
- Do they struggle to solve simple math problems in their head?
- Do they struggle to complete written projects that require details and complex thoughts?
- Do they struggle to keep up with conversation?
- Do they become overwhelmed when too much information is presented at once?
- Do they need more time to make decisions or give answers?
- Do they need to read information more than once for comprehension?
- Do they take longer than expected to get ready in the morning?
- Do they miss nuances in conversation?
- Do they struggle to keep up with other people/kids?
- Do they struggle to grasp subtle social cues?
- Do they struggle with reading fluency skills? Do they fail to complete a reading passage in a certain time or during an exam? Do they have difficulty finishing large reading projects?
- Do they struggle to sustain attention to a task because the information is coming so quickly that they lose track and become "lost?"
- Do they struggle to quickly retrieve information from long-term memory?
- Do they struggle to make decisions regarding everyday tasks, such as deciding what they are going to wear, brushing their teeth, or taking a shower?
- Are they slow at eating and do mealtimes take extended periods of time?
- Do they struggle to complete simple chores, such as taking out the trash?
- Do they struggle with visual processing, such as looking up phone numbers, reading directions, counting out change, or finding an item on a crowded shelf?
- Do they struggle with verbal processing, such as responding to instructions to move themselves or an object or understanding verbal communication and developing a cogent response?

- Do they struggle with motor speed, such as listening to a teacher and taking notes at the same time (slow written output)?
- Do they often appear tired even after being well-rested? Do they appear lazy or unmotivated?
- Do they struggle to participate in classroom discussion?
- Even when they know the right answer, do they hesitate to give it?
- Do they frequently respond with "What?" despite having adequate hearing?

Based on: Braaten & Willoughby (2014).

Observation and Development of Visual Motor Functioning

Fine/Graphomotor Skills

The following table focuses on the development of fine or graphomotor skills that contribute to handwriting. The assessments listed, while not assessing handwriting directly, are the most common tools used by neuropsychologists or occupational therapists to evaluate the fine motor skills necessary for handwriting skills to emerge.

TABLE 5.1 Fine Motor and Graphomotor Skill Development

Age	*Fine/Graphomotor Skills*	*Assessments*
3–4 years	• Able to draw straight vertical and horizontal lines, circles • Able to draw rudimentary likeness of a person	• Beery-Buktenica Developmental Test of Visual-Motor Integration, 6th Edition (Beery VMI) • Bender Visual Motor Gestalt, 2nd Edition (Bender Gestalt II) • NEPSY-II: Design Copying • Wide Range Assessment of Visual Motor Abilities (WRAVMA)
4–5 years	• Able to copy a cross, square, oblique lines	• Beery VMI • Bender Gestalt II • NEPSY-II • WRAVMA
5–6 years	• Able to copy an oblique cross, triangle • Able to copy letters • Able to copy first name • Able to print numbers 1–5	• Beery VMI • Bender Gestalt II • NEPSY-II • WRAVMA • ROCF
6–7 years	• Quality of handwriting improves quickly	• Beery VMI • Bender Gestalt II • NEPSY-II • WRAVMA • ROCF

(continued)

TABLE 5.1 *(continued)*

Age	*Fine/Graphomotor Skills*	*Assessments*
7–8 years	• Improvement in handwriting quality plateaus	• Beery VMI • Bender Gestalt II • NEPSY-II • WRAVMA • ROCF
8–9 years	• Handwriting becomes automatic, organized • Handwriting becomes tool for development of ideas • Speed of handwriting develops in linear fashion	• Beery VMI • Bender Gestalt II • NEPSY-II • WRAVMA • ROCF
9–18 years	• Handwriting continues to develop as a tool for expression	• Beery VMI • Bender Gestalt II • NEPSY-II (up to 16 years) • WRAVMA (up to 17 years) • ROCF

Sources: Beery et al. (2010), Carter (2009), and Feder & Majnemer (2007).

Processing Speed

Within the current context, cognitive efficiency is defined by measures of processing speed. These measures, in turn, are determined by the results of assessments that typically involve scanning complex visual information and organizing motor output, usually in the form of a pencil and paper task (e.g., crossing out a target stimulus within a complex visual array, copying symbols beneath paired numbers in visually dense answer spaces). For additional information about specific tests, see Reinstein and Burau (2014).

Due to a paucity of observational information and research on the development of processing speed in children, the following chart highlights the development of cognitive efficiency in children aged 5 to 18 as measured by two subtests on the Woodcock Johnson Tests of Achievement. The Cross Out test consists of 30 rows with a target stimulus at the left and 19 similar figures to the right. The child places a line through the five of the 19 figures identical to the one at the left. On the Visual Matching test, there are 60 rows, each of which includes six digits, two of which are identical. The child circles the identical digits. On each of the tests, the child is given three minutes to complete as many as possible. The chart also provides information related to processing speed assessments typically performed by psychologists and neuropsychologists. It is important to note that speed of processing can impact fluency in reading, math, and written expression.

TABLE 5.2 Processing Speed Development

Age	*Processing Speed**	*Assessments*
5–6 years	• Approximately 4 correct on Cross Out task • Approximately 6 correct on Visual Matching task	• WPPSI-IV • WISC-V • WJ-IV-COG • Woodcock Johnson IV – Test of Achievement (WJ-IV Ach) • SB-5
6–7 years	• Approximately 8 correct on Cross Out task • Approximately 20 correct on Visual Matching task	• WPPSI-IV • WISC-V • WJ-IV-COG • WJ-IV Ach • SB-5
7–9 years	• Approximately 15 correct on Cross Out task • Approximately 30 correct on Visual Matching task	• WISC-V • WJ-IV-COG • SB-5
10–12 years	• Approximately 20 correct on Cross Out task • Approximately 40 correct on Visual Matching task	• WISC-V • WJ-IV-COG • SB-5
12–14 years	• Approximately 25 correct on Cross Out task • Approximately 45 correct on Visual Matching task	• WISC-V • WJ-IV-COG • SB-5
14–16 years	• Approximately 27 correct on Cross Out task • Approximately 50 correct on Visual Matching task	• WISC-V • WJ-IV-COG • SB-5
16–18 years	• Approximately 28 correct on Cross Out task • Approximately 52 correct on Visual Matching task	• WISC-V • WJ-IV-COG • SB-5

Note: * Approximations of values on the Woodcock Johnson Tests of Achievement Cross Out and Visual Matching tasks derived from Kail and Ferrer (2007) and on the Cross Out task from Ferrer et al. (2013).

Developing Accommodations and Interventions

Once a child's strengths and vulnerabilities in graphomotor skills and processing speed have been identified, accommodations can be put in place and interventions can be made. The following sections indicate specific interventions that can be made to address an individual's emotional needs while integrating a strength-based approach. Individualizing the accommodation or intervention is important. Also, bear in mind the importance of addressing both academic and social/emotional elements of functioning. Furthermore, it is important to remember that all of the following accommodations and strategies are best implemented within the context of a holding environment (Winnicott, 1965) that has a foundation based in the relationship formed between the teacher or specialist and the child.

General Academic Accommodations and Strategies

The following list of accommodations and strategies can be implemented in the classroom. Some of these accommodations can be included in an IEP or 504 plan.

General Graphomotor Accommodations

- Use an alphabet line taped to the desk.
- Allow extended time to complete assignments and reduce the volume of written output.
- Allow opportunities to give oral answers for exercises, quizzes, and tests versus written answers.
- Use word-processing programs with spelling and grammar checks.
- Provide explicit instruction in typing.
- Provide outlines for lectures and class materials to reduce organization load and focus on writing skills.
- Provide a scribe (at student request) for assessments, tests, and exams.
- Reduce amount of writing/pencil work.
- Use highlighting and Post-Its in textbooks and while taking notes.
- Utilize alternative grading system that allows for separate grades for: (1) appearance and mechanics of writing, and (2) content.
- Consult with occupational therapist.
- Teach use of graphic organizers/outlines/mapping skills.
- Teach proofreading skills and allow checklist for proofreading.
- Use tape recorder during lecture.
- Allow frequent breaks during assessment and tests.
- Prompt student to maintain appropriate posture required for writing. Consult with an occupational therapist for posture maintenance strategies.
- Establish preferred seating close to the board or projector.

Graphomotor Writing Accommodations/Modifications

- Use raised line paper.
- Use highlighted paper to distinguish between upper- and lower-case letters.
- Use specialized writing equipment: weighted pencil, vary length and thickness of pencil.
- Highlight or outline areas to be used on worksheets.
- Use a slant board (writing easel).
- Provide lists and simple sentences.
- Allow student to dictate to a teacher or peer.
- Use cloze procedure or fill-in-the-blank for evaluation and early report writing.
- Provide supplemental visual markers on a page and prompt a student where to write and how to organize their work.
- Provide a pencil grip.

Graphomotor Reading Accommodations

- Provide notetaking format.
- Highlight key words or concepts.
- Use guided reading strips to help student keep their place while reading.
- Use one-page summaries or study guides to replace lengthy reading review assignments.
- Use large-print books/font.

Graphomotor Math Accommodations

- Use graph paper to assist in lining up and organizing math problems.
- Enlarge worksheets/assignments for more writing space.
- Allow use of number line.
- Reduce number of practice or test items per page.
- Reduce/avoid having student copy problem sets from text book. Provide student with pre-made corresponding worksheets.
- Allow use of calculator with print-out.
- Allow use of speech-recognition devices, such as a talking tape measure.

General Processing Speed Accommodations

- Allow extra time on assignments and tests.
- Establish predictable schedule and classroom routines.
- Teach time-management strategies.
- Allow access to technology. When checking websites for classroom assignments, have all assignments listed on one site instead of multiple sites.
- Provide a model/example of a completed assignment.
- Use simplified directions and language.
- Break into small manageable chunks: either assign a specific amount of work to complete that is reasonable for that student or assign a timeframe (read for 20 minutes) regardless of the amount of work that is completed.
- Provide extra set of textbooks for home use.
- Provide lectures in advance.
- Provide lecture notes from a peer or teacher.
- Reduce tasks that require multi-tasking.
- Reduce problems on one page.
- Model completed project before student begins.
- Shorten repetitive assignments.
- Provide extended time for tests and assignments.
- Limit amount of time spent on homework and assignments.
- Use cloze procedure.
- Provide word bank.
- Allow sufficient time for student to formulate a response.

- Emphasize accuracy and quality in grading rather than number of completed items.
- Provide individualized or small group test-taking.
- Provide a cue before calling on a student.
- Use timer to increase self-monitoring of output and speed of completion.

Processing Speed Reading Accommodations/Strategies

- Use audiobooks or books on tape.
- Allow access to word processor.
- Provide copies of notes, formatted with only key words needing to be added.
- Provide high-interest books at student's reading level.
- Provide resource folder.
- Model fluent reading by reading aloud.
- Use choral reading.
- Practice sight words using flash cards.
- Use repeated reading of text.
- Preview reading material.

Processing Speed Writing Accommodations

- Allow use of word-processing programs.
- Allow use of speech-recognition software.
- Emphasize quality not quantity.
- Use graphic organizers.

Processing Speed Math Accommodations

- Frequently repeat facts.
- Use computerized math programs that focus on increasing the automaticity of math facts.
- Use flash cards to precut math facts.

Addressing Visual Motor Functioning

As illustrated in the opening vignette, difficulty with VMI skills, like with many of the neuropsychological functional domains, can have a dual impact on a student's development: it impacts their learning directly (difficulty with handwriting) and it can impact their sense of self as a student and overall self-perception. Studies have drawn direct connections between VMI development and performance in math and written expression (Carlson et al., 2013). In general, motor development is linked to cognitive development, and a variety of developmental disorders can correlate with motor difficulties or they can occur independently of cognitive difficulties (Davis et al., 2011). Careful assessment can tease out aspects of motor functioning and cognitive functioning to develop treatment plans and make appropriate and specific accommodations. It is also important to note that, like with other functional domains, culture and experience impact the development of VMI skills (Lim et al., 2015).

In the following sections, specific concerns and interventions regarding graphomotor skills and processing speed as they relate to academic and social/emotional development are discussed. Overall treatment of VMI skills is within the purview of occupational therapy. When developing interventions and strategies to promote development of these skills, consulting with an occupational therapist can bring deeper understanding and better application of interventions. However, several games and toys naturally promote the development of VMI skills and are briefly listed here.

Games/Activities for VMI Development

Make a salt or clay tray and have the individual draw or write in the tray using their fingers or a golf tee; play with soap foam or shaving cream; use popsicle sticks to imitate or make shapes and letters; use a peg board or Lite-Brite to make shapes and letters; string colored beads; make paper chains; build with Legos, blocks and Lincoln Logs; use sidewalk chalk (with stencils); play games with balloons; coloring activities; cooking activities such as making ants on a log that require the individual to place small food items onto a larger food item; Quiddler; Bop It; Stare!; Rush Hour; Quirkle; and Blockus.

INTERVENTIONS FOR GRAPHOMOTOR SKILLS

Students who struggle with developing handwriting skills are often diagnosed with dysgraphia, a term referring to non-efficient handwriting and a specific disorder of written expression (Deuel, 1994). Graphomotor difficulties, along with issues related to language, attention, spatial ordering, sequential ordering, and memory, contribute to dysgraphia. Beginning in kindergarten, handwriting tasks frequently occur in every grade (Marr et al., 2001). As you have seen in the list of accommodations, access to keyboards and typing instruction is often an accommodation for individuals with graphomotor difficulties. It is important to be aware that typing is a fine motor skill and, while it requires different skills than handwriting, it can still pose a problem for individuals with general fine motor difficulties (Niles-Campbell et al., 2008). Targeted intervention often occurs with an occupational therapist in either individual or small group remediation and in consultation to the classroom.

Games/Activities that Promote Graphomotor Skills

Drawing; step-by-step drawing books; coloring books; completing simple mazes; connect-the-dots activities; origami; playing with play dough or clay; construction toys such as Lego and blocks; tracing patterns and shapes; channeling activities (drawing a line between two guiding lines that are wide enough and straight enough for the individual's level of graphomotor development); copying activities; use of stencils; Magna Doodle; and use of different writing/drawing surfaces such as a chalk board, whiteboard, or sand tray.

ACADEMIC

There are a variety of ways in which graphomotor development impacts academic performance. Aside from the difficulty with handwriting, the lack of automaticity disrupts the simultaneous act of composition (Graham, 1990; Scardamalia et al., 1982). More demands can be put on memory and attentional capacity, constraining higher-level cognitive processes required for composition (Berninger & Graham, 1998; Jones & Christensen, 1999). If the act of transferring ideas and plans to the page is slowed by handwriting, the student may forget the idea altogether (Graham & Weintraub, 1996). Furthermore, it has been suggested that teachers give higher marks for papers and assignments that are neatly written. Therefore, penmanship may influence the perception of a student's competency (Rosenblum et al., 2003). With all these factors at play, students may become frustrated and avoid writing work altogether, resulting in delayed or arrested writing development and less effort put forth towards planning of a composition or revision of their work (McCutchen, 1996).

Math – The way in which dysgraphia impacts math seems less obvious, but writing, drawing, and other fine motor activities can impact a student's ability to complete math work. Inconsistent spacing between numbers and symbols can make it difficult for students to complete operations such as long division or track information in algebra equations. The accidental omission of numbers, letters, and words can lead to calculation mistakes. Students may struggle to copy numbers and formulas from the board. Tasks that involve drawing (such as making charts and graphs) may be difficult. The extra effort these students make related to their graphomotor skills can result in decreased cognitive capacity for organizing their thoughts, completing mental math and working through various steps of math problems (Cherry, 2016).

ENVIRONMENTAL CONSIDERATIONS

- Provide adaptive technology as appropriate with consultation.
- Provide adaptive writing materials such as raised line paper, slant boards, and different types of writing implements (pencils of different girth, reloadable pencils to prevent heavy pressure, and pencil grips) with consultation by an occupational therapist.

OTHER SERVICES

- Occupational therapy.

Interventions for Processing Speed

Many of the accommodations for slow processing speed are related to the amount of time a student takes to complete an assignment. In addition to allowing extra time, intervention can include teaching students time-management skills. This includes specifically teaching the student to tell time, estimate how long a task will take (task analysis), and work within a specific allotted time (Lemov, 2015). It is important to teach children with slow processing speed how their pace is the same or different from others and how to pace themselves, and especially important to do so without shaming or embarrassing them. This can be done by teaching concepts about time management in playful game-like ways in which there is not a winner based on how fast an activity is completed. See the Chapter 5 Appendix for specific activities on teaching time management. Some of these activities can be used as math curriculum depending on the grade level and state curriculum.

SOCIAL/EMOTIONAL

Individuals with slow processing can struggle socially, but this is not always the case. At any developmental level, slow processing plays a role in comprehending and responding to verbal, non-verbal, and motoric interactions. Some ways in which slow processing speed impacts social interactions include (Braaten & Willoughby, 2014):

- They may take longer to pick up on social cues and misunderstand or miss the point of the interaction.
- They require extra time to develop a response, so interactions can feel stilted or awkward.
- During pretend play or games, they lose track of what is happening. This may result in their own frustration or frustration for their peers.
- They can be disorganized when telling stories. As a result, peers lose interest and move on to another activity.
- They are frequently late to appointments and meetings as a result of poor time management. As a result, peers are frustrated.
- Reactions to jokes or sarcasm are delayed. This can appear awkward and confusing to peers.
- When working collaboratively in groups, slow work performance can be frustrating to peers.

As we saw with Anthony in the opening vignette, slow processing speed can also impact a child's emotional well-being, which in turn can lead to a host of behavioral issues. Individuals with slow processing speed often experience low self-esteem, depression, and anxiety. In children, this can manifest through irritability, oppositional behaviors, inappropriately boastful comments, perfectionistic tendencies, overreactions to small issues or problems, difficulty eating or sleeping, procrastination, difficulty with change, social isolation, school refusal, stomachaches and headaches, lethargy, hypervigilance, and withdrawal. Understanding that a cognitive vulnerability may be at the root of an emotional and/or behavioral issue is an important step in building empathy and compassion for a child whose behaviors may be very difficult to be around. Recognizing this issue and putting appropriate supports in place can be an important step in ameliorating behavioral issues and addressing the individual's needs.

Some individuals with processing speed issues can benefit from learning specific social skills that promote connectivity and keeping pace with peers. Teaching whole-body listening (Truesdale, 1990) or active listening (Gordon & Burch, 1974) can help a child or teen who gets lost in social situations to persevere when lost and show peers and teachers they are interested, and help them to attend. These approaches teach individuals skills for attending and listening versus hearing and how to display to peers through body language that they are attending. Other processing disabilities can make it difficult for them to express typical cues that they are attending. For example, some individuals with visual processing difficulties may struggle to engage in typical eye contact when engaged in conversation. For this reason, some may struggle to develop all the expected active listening skills and may need extra support and accommodations.

Games that Utilize Processing Speed

Taboo; Scattergories; Simplexity; Set; Slamwhich; Quitch; Blink; Pix Mix; Spot It; Rat-a-Tat Cat; Rock; 7 ate 9; Bop It; and Dance Dance Revolution.

ACADEMIC

Behaviors resulting from slow processing speed can impact a student's ability to access the curriculum. Underlying these emotional reactions to impaired processing speed are ways in which processing speed impacts learning.

Reading – Several studies have been conducted in an attempt to understand the role that processing speed plays in the development of reading skills. Reading is a complex ability that requires several neural systems to work in harmony (Reinstein & Burau, 2014). Parsing out the exact role that processing speed plays in the development of this skill has proven to be difficult because of the various processing abilities that impact reading development. It is known that children with oral language weaknesses (C. A. Miller et al., 2001, 2006) and word reading or reading fluency weaknesses (Wolf & Bowers, 1999) also display reduced processing speed. It has also been demonstrated that processing speed contributes to Rapid Automatized Naming (RAN – the ability to rapidly name highly familiar visual stimuli) but other cognitive processes also contribute (Kirby et al., 2010). Also, processing speed does not consistently predict broad measures of language ability (Poll et al., 2013).

Math – Processing speed (along with working memory) has been shown to impact development of early numeracy math cognitive tasks (numbers and counting) (Geary et al., 2007). Processing speed has also been linked to arithmetic calculations and computational fluency with basic facts. It has been linked to math skills that require automaticity, such as fact retrieval (Fuchs et al., 2005; Geary, 2004). While working memory is often studied alongside processing speed, studies indicate that processing speed is a strong predictor of arithmetic competence (Bull & Johnston, 1997) and may be a stronger predictor than working memory (Fuchs et al., 2005).

ENVIRONMENTAL CONSIDERATIONS

- Provide an environment that is free of clutter.
- Hang analog clocks.

OTHER SERVICES

- Executive functioning coaching tutoring.
- Individual or group therapy (for social skills development or for developing an understanding of their learning style).

Chapter 5 Appendix: Visual Motor Functioning Interventions

GRAPHOMOTOR SKILLS: ACTIVITIES TO PROMOTE DEVELOPMENT

Goal: Promote the development of graphomotor skills through low-stress activities that strengthen hand muscles, pencil grasp, and visual tracking.

Materials: Various worksheets that allow the students to trace, connect dots, or do mazes.

Directions: During breaks or when students finish their assigned work, provide various worksheets (that can contain themes of interest or seasonal themes) which motivate students to engage in activities promoting the development of graphomotor skills.

Adaptation: These worksheets could also relate to curriculum themes.

Worksheets based on Terapeut u Kuci, http://terapeut-u-kuci.com/.

Tracing Activity

Name: ______________________________

Trace the line that connects the matching shapes, using a highlighter or marker that matches the shape.

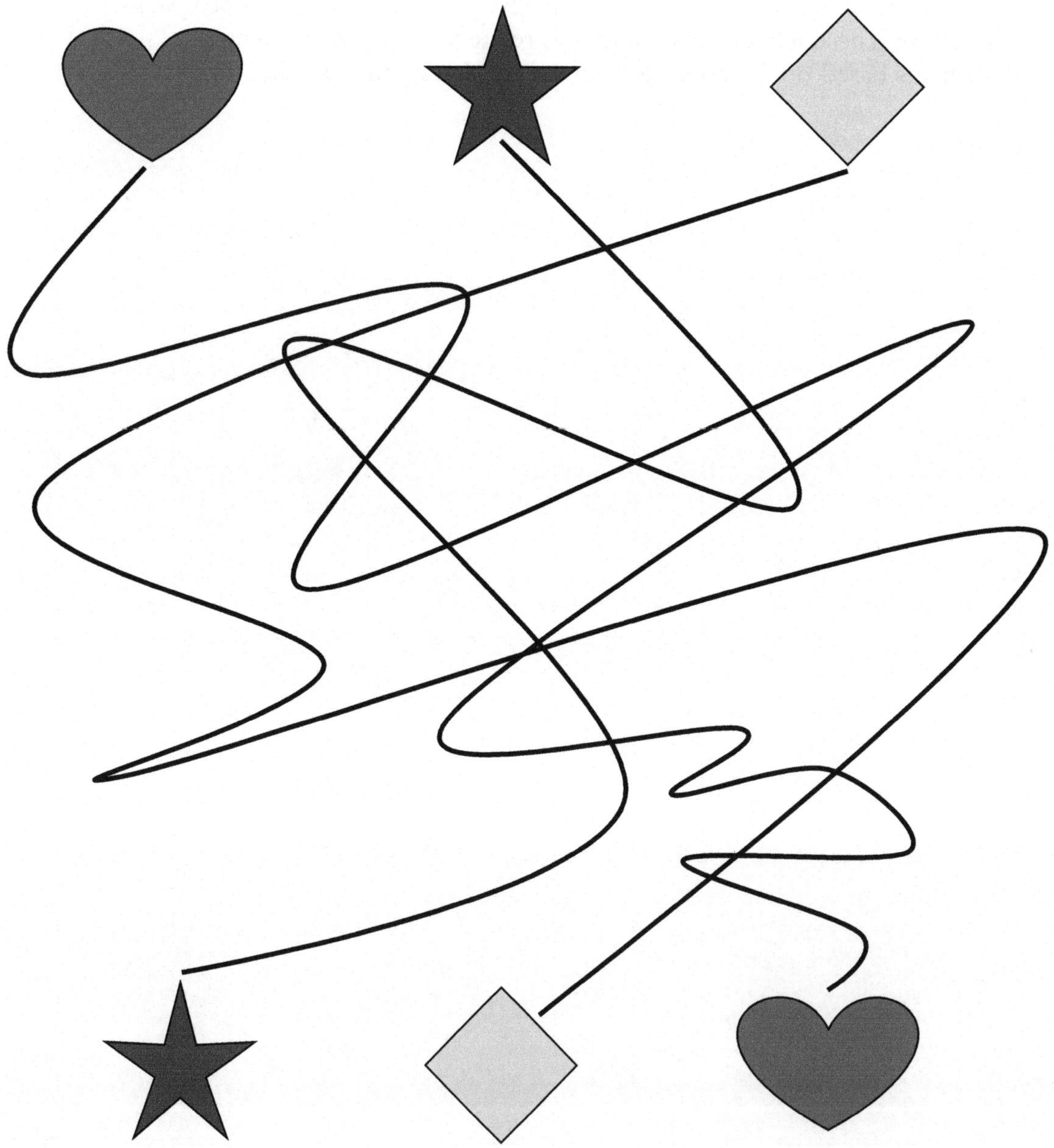

Connect the Dots

Name: ____________________________

Draw a line to connect the dots.

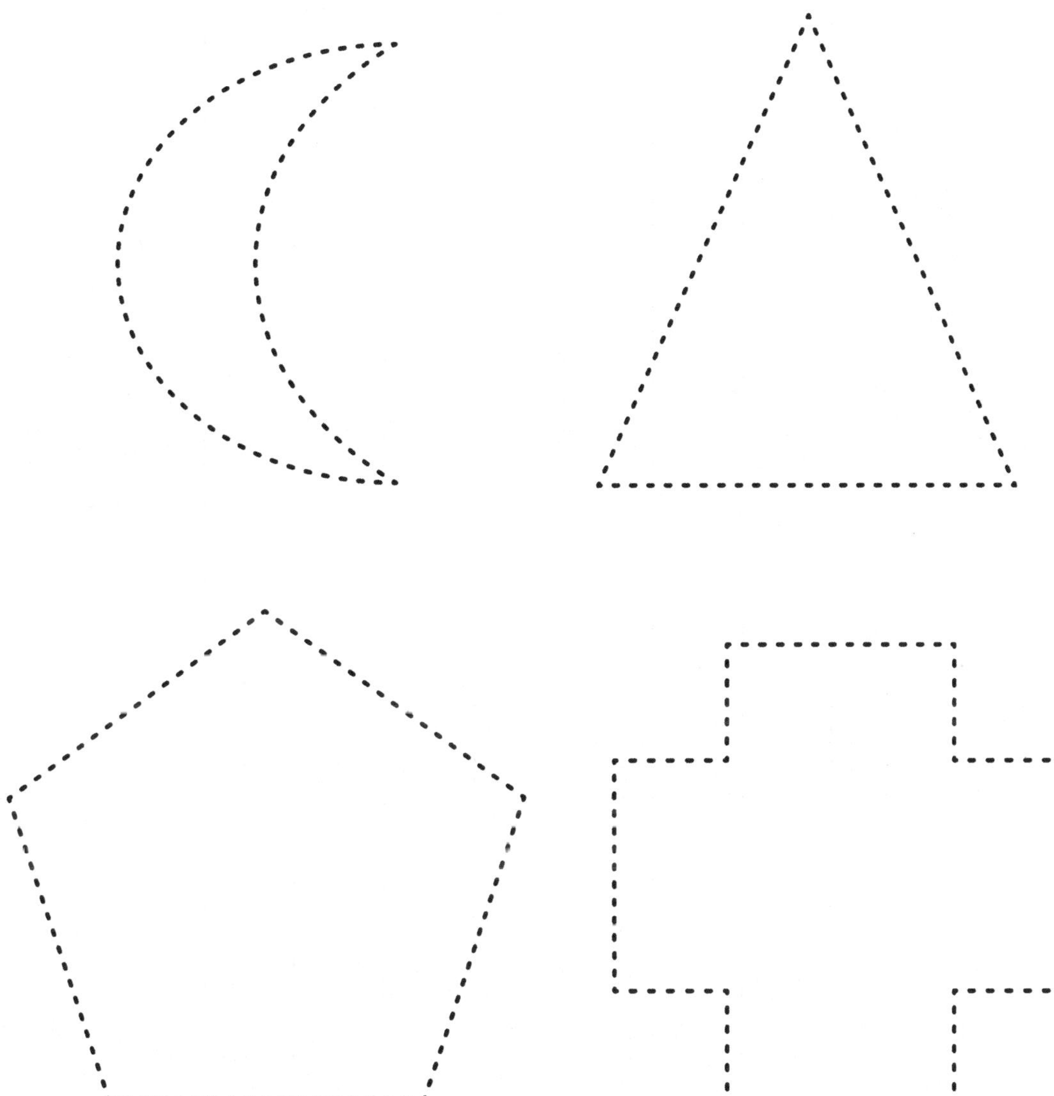

Maze Activity

Name: ___________________________

Use a pencil to help the girl find her way home.

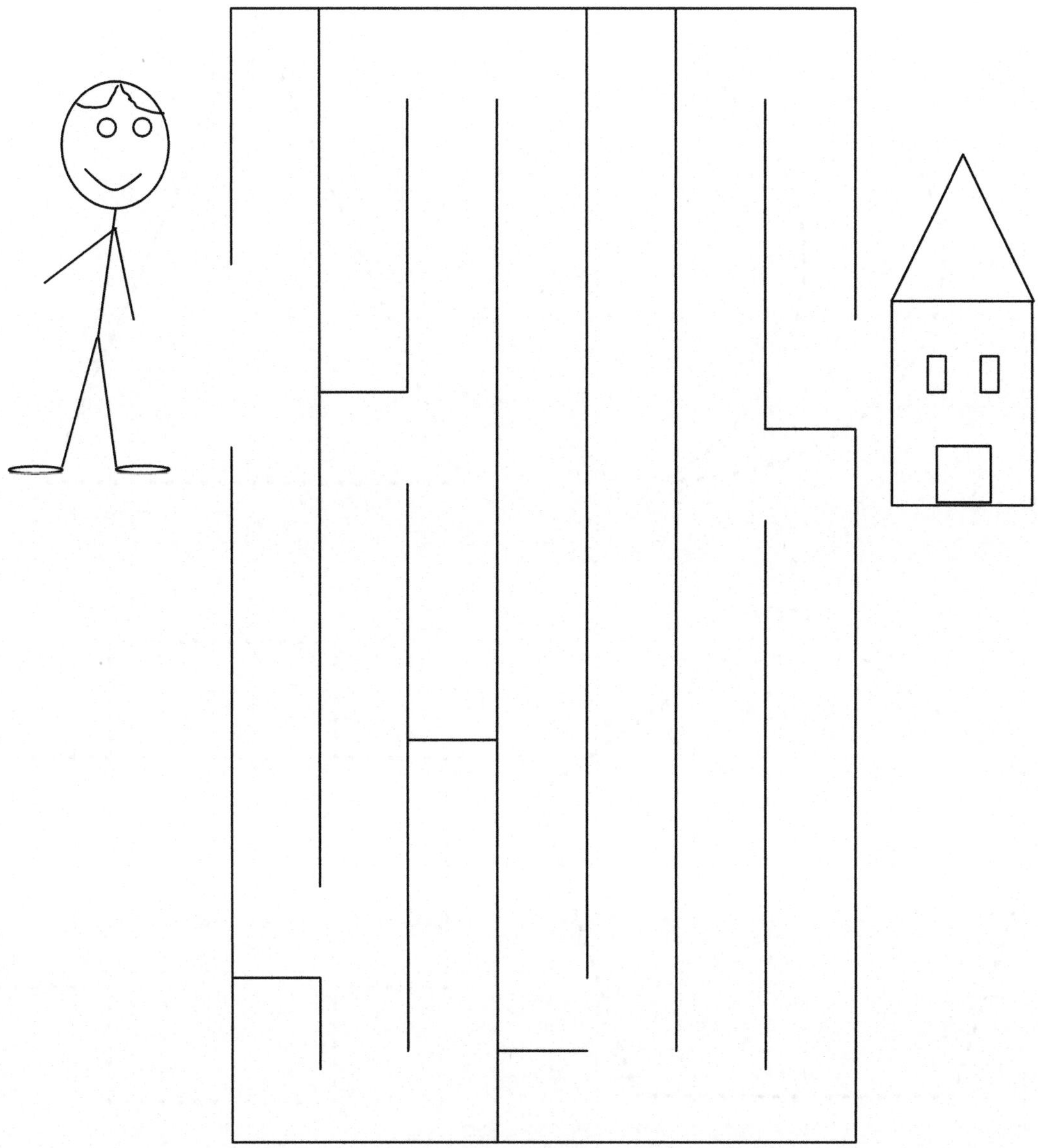

GRAPHOMOTOR SKILLS: PROMOTING HANDWRITING DEVELOPMENT

Goal: Motivate students to properly space between words, making their writing more legible.

Material: Small stickers (smiley face stickers or stickers that align with their interests, such as hearts, sports balls, or flowers), paper, pencil.

Directions: During a writing activity such as a free-write, journal, or handwriting lesson (depending on age and grade), or while copying sentences, instruct the students to use small stickers in between every word they write. Allow them to choose a preferred sticker. Demonstrate how it should look to have stickers between each word. If the students are not motivated by this alone, provide a small incentive for using a designated number of stickers. For example, if they use 10 small stickers to space words, they will then earn a large sticker for the cover of their journal, extra play time, or a small task they enjoy.

PROCESSING SPEED: TEACHING TIME ESTIMATION AND TASK ANALYSIS

Goal: Heighten student awareness of how long it takes to complete various tasks. Develop skills in recognizing how many steps are required to complete a task.

Materials: Stopwatch, Task Analysis and Time Estimation Sheet.

Directions: Explain to the students that over the course of the week, as a group, you will be studying time estimation and task analysis. The project is all about learning about time, how quickly time can pass, and how long it can take to do different activities. Clarify with the group that it is *not* about racing and seeing who can do something the fastest, but on developing the ability to make a good guess about *how long* it will take to do different tasks.

Ask the students what types of activities they already know how long it will take them to do or if they have ever measured how long it takes to do something before (races in gym class or in a sport, the length of a TV show, etc.). Generate a list of these activities, noting that some take a short time, a medium time, and a long time.

Ask the students about their favorite songs. Have them research how long each of their favorite songs are, noting that even though the time is different they are all considered to be a song.

Introduce the Time Estimation and Task Analysis Sheet. Explain to the students that throughout the week this will be used to guess and measure how long it takes to do various activities. Choose a simple and well-known classroom routine. Using the stopwatch, time the students and complete the worksheet together, including the steps to the classroom routine. You can have the students intentionally vary the rate at which they complete the worksheet (fast speed, slow-mo and regular) to demonstrate a bodily sense of how it feels to go at the regular pace.

Finally, have the students generate a list of tasks (routines, play, and academic) that will be analyzed as a group over the course of the week. Once the procedure is well known, assign the students some tasks that they can analyze at home (making the bed, biking to a friend's house, etc.).

Adaptations:

- Students could independently complete individual worksheets or they could be completed as a group.
- If students struggle with graphomotor skills, type out the various steps, adding some extraneous steps for them to include, and ask the students to put the steps in the correct order.

Based on: Newell (2008).

Task Analysis and Time Estimation Sheet

Task: ______________________________

Estimated Time for Task Completion	→	
Actual Time to Complete	→	
Task Difference Between Estimate and Actual	→	

Steps:

1. ______________________________
2. ______________________________
3. ______________________________
4. ______________________________
5. ______________________________
6. ______________________________
7. ______________________________
8. ______________________________
9. ______________________________
10. ______________________________
11. ______________________________

PROCESSING SPEED: COMPARING TIME ESTIMATES AND TASK ACTIVITIES

Goal: Develop time estimation skills and compare various task lengths.

Materials: Different colored pencils or markers, graph paper, timer, stopwatch, or clock.

Directions: After having students complete the Task Analysis and Time Estimation activity, continue to build their knowledge of time management by making a bar graph. Take the actual and estimated time for each activity. Teaching the students about the X axis and Y axis and have them create a bar graph that visually displays the various activities, how long each one took, and how close their estimates were. Depending on grade level, this can be used as part of their math curriculum.

Adaptation: Bar graphs can also be represented using blocks and manipulatives such as Unifix Cubes. This works well for students who do best when engaged with hands-on materials.

Based on: Newhall (2008).

PROCESSING SPEED: PROVIDING SOCIAL SUPPORT

- Simplify social situations. When grouping students, make groups smaller so there are not as many people, comments, and ideas for the child to keep track of.
- Provide guidance in social situations. Have conversations with the individual, teaching them to politely request other people to slow down their rate of speech or repeat their ideas. For example, "Give me a second please. I need time to think."
- Provide scripts for how to ask for clarification ("What did you mean when you said that?" "I'm sorry I didn't get all that, can you repeat it please?").
- Cue the individual to read non-verbal as well as verbal information. Know if they have a visual or auditory strength and help them rely on it to decipher social situations.
- Teach active listening.
- Help the individual recognize their coping strategy when they are overwhelmed by fast social situations. Help them recognize if it is a helpful strategy or causing more problems. Try not to overwhelm the individual with negative messages, and point out what they are doing correctly.
- During play dates or social interactions, be sure to closely monitor the transition into play and give space as appropriate. Provide scaffolding (explain social cues and situations) as necessary. When possible, allow the children to be independent.
- Preview new situations (such as field trips, sports activities, new academic activities, and games). Provide vocabulary, set expectations, allow time for questions and conversation, and provide scripts they can rely on in the moment. Potentially pair the individual with another student they trust and like.

Based on: Braaten & Willoughby (2014).

PROCESSING SPEED: TEACHING ACTIVE LISTENING

Goal: Develop understanding of hearing versus listening and its importance in social interactions. Begin to develop active listening skills.

Materials: Paper and markers (or preferred drawing material).

Directions: Tell the students you will be doing an experiment to learn about hearing versus listening. Have students brainstorm what they think the difference might be. Tell them that you will go into different environments and find what they can listen to. If possible, take students on a walk outside. (If not possible, this activity can be done in a classroom or in another room in the building.) While outside, ask the class to be still and hear with their ears and listen to the sound of being outside. Ask the students to name what they are hearing and ask them if they have heard it before. Go into different rooms within the school and ask them to hear and listen. Ask them what they had to do differently in their bodies to help them listen to the different environments. Upon returning to the classroom, have students draw one of the environments the class explored, highlighting the different sounds.

Make the connection that sometimes when we are with people, it can be easy to just hear but not listen, or that listening can be hard if the other person is too fast, slow, loud, or quiet, uses strange words, and so on. Ask students to list all the things that make it hard for them to listen to another person. Ask the class which one of the items on the list they would like to develop strategies for managing so that they can be active listeners if their friends engage in one of the difficult behaviors.

Adaptation: In another lesson, if age appropriate, read *Whole Body Listening Larry at Home!* and *Whole Body Listening Larry at School!* (Sautter & Wilson, 2016). These books encourage students to look at the person talking, hear what is being said, keep a quiet mouth, have still hands in their lap or by their sides, keep feet on the floor and keep them still, face the person who is speaking, use their brain to think about the person who is speaking, and use their head to care about what they say. The books can then be used as a format to practice various listening skills and body language.

Based on: Truesdale (1990).

PROCESSING SPEED: PROVIDING EMOTIONAL AND BEHAVIORAL SUPPORT

Goal: Support underlying cognitive vulnerabilities that result in social, emotional, and behavioral difficulties.

- Designate a person in the school environment that the student trusts and can speak to/be with when feeling overwhelmed or anxious.
- Frequently and appropriately praise the individual for a job well done. If their behaviors are difficult, this can feel hard to do in an authentic and sincere way. Cultivate compassion for the child's vulnerabilities.
- Use positive reinforcements versus negative consequences to improve behavior in the classroom.
- Attempt to avoid social situations that might cause the individual embarrassment.
- Preview new activities and set clear expectations.
- Provide "jobs" or "tasks" that the individual can successfully complete within the classroom environment. This promotes feelings of success, allows meaningful contribution to the classroom, and allows other students to see the individual as successful. Tailor the jobs to the student's strengths and interests.
- Engage in clear and frequent communication between home, school and all personnel working with the individual.

Based on: Braaten & Willoughby (2014).

PROCESSING SPEED: MATH – DIFFERENT WAYS TO MEASURE PASSAGE OF TIME

Goals: Identify the various ways in which the passage of time is measured, and identify an effective strategy and preference for how to measure time spent on various activities.

Materials: Analog clock, digital clock, sand glass, time timer, liquid timer, stopwatch, and time tracker.

Directions: Have a conversation with the students about the different ways to measure time. Develop a display in which an analog clock, digital clock, and sand glass timer measure the same unit of time (preferably a short time for the purpose of demonstration). Brainstorm the different activities and places in which different ways to measure time might be used (playing board games, timing a race, time to complete homework). Throughout the day, use the different measuring techniques to demonstrate how they can be used for various activities. When students are doing quiet classroom work, allow them to choose a method of time measurement and put it on their desk(s).

PROCESSING SPEED: READING – DISCUSSING TIME/TIME COLLAGE

Goal: Explore the language we use in discussing time. Develop more comfort with a concept that may have negative associations. Integrate potential reading standards into the discussion about time.

Materials: Heavy paper for collaging, glue, images of different ways to measure time (analog clock, sundials, hourglass, sunrise and sunsets, etc.), printed phrases about time using different fonts/colors, scissors, stickers, other collage materials, printout with different definitions of the word "time," printout of idioms and common time-related sayings.

Directions: Start the lesson by asking students to brainstorm the different ways that time is discussed throughout the day (see examples below). Note that the way the word "time" is used is the same in each example. Hand out the printout containing all the different definitions of the word "time" and note that it is a noun, adjective and verb. Ask the students what different emotions/feelings may be associated with time. Write the emotions/feelings on the board. Hand out the list of idioms and sayings about time. Ask the students to read through the list and make an image using the collaging materials that reflects how the word "time" is used in the English language. Display the completed collages.

Adaptations:

- If students have not learned about idioms, adapt the lesson to teach these concepts.
- Break this lesson into smaller segments (define time then introduce the list of metaphors and idioms).
- Present only a few of the definitions and idioms to prevent overwhelming the students.
- Rephrase time definitions to students' reading level.

Different phrases used when discussing time:

- What time is it?
- It's time to pack up.
- You're wasting time.
- Do we have time for that?
- It's time for music class.
- Be sure to hand in your work on time.
- We're out of time today.
- It's lunchtime.
- If I have to tell you one more time . . .

Definitions of Time:

NOUN

1. The system of those sequential relations that any event has to any other, as past, present, or future; indefinite and continuous duration regarded as that in which events succeed one another.
2. Duration regarded as belonging to the present life as distinct from the life to come or from eternity.

3. A system or method of measuring or reckoning the passage of time: mean time; apparent time; etc.
4. A limited period or interval, as between two successive events: a long time.
5. A particular period considered as distinct from other periods: Youth is the best time of life.
6. Often, times. For example: prehistoric times; in Lincoln's time; a sign of the times; how times have changed; hard times; a time of war.

ADJECTIVE

1. Of, relating to, or showing the passage of time.
2. (Of an explosive device) containing a clock so that it will detonate at the desired moment: a time bomb.
3. Of or relating to purchases on the installment plan, or with payment postponed.

VERB (USED WITH OBJECT), TIMED, TIMING.

1. To measure or record the speed, duration or rate of: to time a race.
2. To fix the duration of: the test was timed for 15 minutes.
3. To regulate (a train, clock, etc.) as to time.
4. To appoint or choose the moment or occasion for; schedule: he timed the attack perfectly.

VERB (USED WITHOUT OBJECT), TIMED, TIMING.

1. To keep time sound or move in unison.

Source: *Time*. In Merriam-Webster (2016).

Time Idioms

Against time – in an effort to finish something within a limited period: We worked against time to get out the newspaper.

Ahead of time – before the time due; early: The building was completed ahead of time.

At one time – once; in a former time: At one time, they owned a restaurant. At the same time; at once: They all try to talk at one time.

At the same time – nevertheless; yet: I'd like to try, but at the same time I'm a little afraid.

Beat my (or someone's) time – to compete or win, prevail over a rival: I ran hard and fast to try and beat my previous time.

Behind the times – old-fashioned; dated: These attitudes are behind the times.

Metaphors, Proverbs, and Sayings about Time

- Time heals all wounds (Geoffrey Chaucer).
- A stitch in time saves nine (proverb).
- Better late than never (Le Hsun).
- Take time for all things. Great haste makes waste (Benjamin Franklin).
- Time and tide wait for no man (William Bradford).
- Here today, gone tomorrow (John Calvin).
- Time flies (proverb).
- To everything there is a season; and a time to every purpose under heaven (The Bible).

–6–

Social/Emotional Functioning Interventions

Introduction

As we consider social/emotional functioning in this chapter, we are doing so within the context of relationships. Thus, we are not only taking into account a child's emotional development but his or her social development as well. Therefore, the following discussion, description of development, and consideration of interventions will encompass both.

In Chapter 1, we discussed the work of Donald Winnicott (1965) and his concepts of the natural unfolding of the developmental process, the "good enough" mother and the holding environment. We also examined the work of John Bowlby (1988) and his theory of attachment. But how do these conceptualizations of a child's social and emotional development manifest as she ages and, furthermore, how are they measured as a means to implement strategies and interventions that support her growth? While we have found Winnicott's ideas to be of very significant heuristic value and to have guided all of our work with children, to our knowledge his concepts have not been operationalized in a manner that lends them to quantitative study. Bowlby's theory of attachment, however, has been studied extensively, initially by researchers such as Mary Ainsworth and her colleagues (1978) and subsequently by a host of child development researchers (e.g., Main & Solomon, 1986).

Ainsworth (1978) developed a research paradigm that she designated the Infant Strange Situation, in which a child's behavior in relationship to his or her parent was observed after separation and upon reunion in a strange or novel laboratory environment. She and subsequent researchers identified four classes of attachment behaviors that, without intervention, can persist throughout a child's life and into adulthood. A child with a **secure** attachment misses a parent during separation and greets her parent actively, often initiating physical contact upon reunion. A child with an **avoidant** pattern of attachment fails to cry on separation and ignores the parent upon reunion. A child with a **resistant or ambivalent** attachment pattern may be distressed even before separation, may seem angry or passive, and fails to take comfort in the parent upon reunion. Lastly, a child with a **disorganized/disoriented** attachment pattern appears disorganized even with the parent present and fails to engage the parent upon reunion. These attachment patterns, developed early in life, determine a child's "internal working model of attachment" (Bowlby, 1988) and impact the manner in which a child is or is not able to make use of subsequent relationships. It is also important to note that disruptions in attachment may stem from factors originating in the child's genetic makeup or prenatal experience. A neurologically compromised child may be born into an environment that is not "good enough" through no fault of the parents: an environment that is not an adequate match for the specific needs of a child but which would otherwise be sufficient for the natural unfolding of the developmental process of a child without those needs.

Nevertheless, how might one conceptualize behavior that may be based in a disruption of the developmental process because of a disruption in relationship? Research has focused on two dimensions of behavior that reflect underlying emotional disturbance. **Externalizing problems** such as aggression, oppositionality, property violations (lying, cruelty to animals) or status violations (substance abuse, running away) and **internalizing problems** such as withdrawal, anxiety, fearfulness, and depression are correlated with temperament, home environment, maternal depression, sociodemographics, and cognitive factors (Fanti & Henrich, 2010), all of which can profoundly affect a child's emotional and relational development. Furthermore, there is an extensive array of literature on the relationship between attachment groups and externalizing and internalizing behaviors. For example, Finnegan et al. (1996) found that for both genders, externalizing problems in middle childhood were predicted by an avoidant coping style while for boys internalizing problems were predicted by an ambivalent coping style. Moss et al. (1998) reported that school-age attachment classifications predicted teacher-reported behavior problems with insecure groups more likely to manifest both externalizing and internalizing behavioral difficulties than with the secure group.

However, the nature of subsequent relationships and the potential for those relationships to influence and change a maladaptive internal working model suggests that intervention can improve an individual's outcome (Main & Solomon, 1986). In fact, Buyse et al. (2008) found that the emotional support of teachers provided a protective effect for kindergarten children with high levels of externalizing or internalizing behaviors. The importance of the teacher–child relationship within the context of attachment and behavior has been demonstrated for children in upper grades as well (Verschueren, 2015).

Observing Social/Emotional Functioning

Recognizing behaviors that relate to attachment style, internalizing symptoms, and externalizing symptoms can be an important skill. It is important to note that developmental age can impact the manifestation of internalizing and externalizing symptoms. For example, internalizing symptoms are associated with depression, but in young children depression can be expressed through irritability, agitation, and tantrums versus the more traditional adult presentation of withdrawal, hopelessness, and isolation. It is important to note that a child intermittently demonstrating one or two of the listed behaviors does not necessarily mean that there is a serious underlying disturbance in attachment. Rather, it is a pattern of some combination of a number of these behaviors or the intensity of one or two of the more serious ones observed over time which may suggest a need for intervention.

Possible Indications of Internalizing Symptoms

CHILDREN

- Do they pretend to be sick or frequently complain of aches and pains with no medical explanation?
- Do they refuse to go to school?
- Do they cling to parents or caregivers?
- Do they worry that parents or caregivers may die?
- Do they struggle to concentrate?
- Are they easily irritated by peers?
- Do they have physical characteristics of being sad or depressed? Do they frequently cry?
- Do they struggle to plan or organize beyond what is developmentally appropriate?
- Do they have a tendency to give up on a task before completing it?
- Does their academic work appear to be below the performance level you believe they are capable of? Why?
- Are they extremely sensitive to criticism?
- Do they struggle to follow directions even though they are trying to?
- Do they become mute in certain situations but display full ability to communicate verbally in other settings?
- Do they often ask to see the nurse or go to the bathroom excessively?
- Do they require extra support to make transitions?
- Do they struggle to keep their hands and feet to themselves?
- How well do they tolerate changes in routine?
- Do they disrupt the schoolwork of other children?
- Do they use things that belong to others without permission?
- Do they appear to overreact to stressful situations?
- Do they make up stories about their lives that are clearly grandiose lies?
- Are they able to accurately describe their feelings?

ADOLESCENTS

- Do they sulk and make negative comments or have a negative attitude?
- Do they act grouchy?
- Do they complain about feeling misunderstood?
- Do they seclude themselves or isolate themselves from others beyond being shy or introverted?
- Are they overly argumentative?
- Do they express issues with self-esteem or self-worth?
- Do they often make self-deprecating comments?
- Are there attendance issues?
- Do they often complain of boredom or do they not have any interests?
- Is there a marked reduction of pleasure in activities they once enjoyed?
- Do they display an increase in risk-taking behaviors that are beyond what is developmentally appropriate?
- Do they perform well on tests or essays, but when called on in class have difficulty expressing their knowledge?
- What type of leadership role do they play? None? An inappropriate role (class clown or rallying other kids against the teacher)? Are they part of various social groups?
- Do they ever start or spread rumors?
- How often do they break the rules?
- Are they able to accurately describe their feelings?
- How do they respond to new teachers? How do they respond to teachers they have known a long time?
- Do they struggle to follow directions or pay attention?
- Do they take things or use things without permission?
- Do they seek attention while doing schoolwork?
- Do they attempt to manipulate others?
- Do they hurt other people on purpose?

Based on: Stephens (2016); Crundwell & Killu (2007); and Reynolds & Kamphaus (2015).

POSSIBLE INDICATIONS OF EXTERNALIZING SYMPTOMS

- Are they frequently irritable?
- Are they often non-compliant? Do they appear to intentionally refuse to follow directions?
- Do they frequently display disruptive behavior? Do they interrupt classroom lessons and routines?
- Are they prone to having extensive and violent tantrums?
- Do they pester other individuals?
- Do they display explosive behavior, moving quickly from calm to aggressive or violent?
- Do they engage in dangerous behavior such as breaking items, stealing things or destroying property?
- Do they use aggression to achieve a goal?

- Do they hurt other children or animals?
- Do they exclude other children from social groups? Do they call other children nasty names or slander others?
- Do they show tendencies toward lying and cheating?
- Do they struggle to maintain attention for long periods of time?
- Do they have difficulty staying on one topic?
- Are they often restless? Do they struggle to sit still?
- Are they easily distracted?

Based on: Liu (2004).

Observation and Development of Social/Emotional Functioning

In the table below, social/emotional development is traced from preschool through high school in respect to what one might expect to observe within a particular developmental timeframe. Assessment tools relevant to that developmental stage are listed as well.

TABLE 6.1 Social/Emotional Development

Age	*Social/Emotional Milestones*	*Assessments*
Preschool	• Increased ability to control emotions (fewer emotional outbursts) • Increased frustration tolerance • Increased ability to delay gratification • Understanding of right/wrong concepts • Rudimentary sense of self develops • Self-esteem based on opinions of significant others • Play is cooperative, imaginative, turn-taking • Seeks to please adults • Developing conscience; feel guilty when disobeying; simplistic idea of good/bad	• Children's Apperception Test – Animals (CAT) – ages 3–10 • Behavior Assessment System for Children, Third Edition (BASC-3) – ages 2–18 • Achenbach System of Empirically-Based Assessment (ASEBA) – ages 1:6–18 • House–Tree–Person (HTP) • Draw a Person (DAP) • Kinetic Family Drawing (KFD)
School-age	• Develops alternative strategies to dealing with frustration and expressing feelings • Attempts to regulate self-conscious emotions (e.g., embarrassment) • Increased awareness of multiple emotions toward same person • Increased sensitivity to others' opinions about himself/herself • Self-esteem increases based on own ability to produce and perform	• CAT • Children's Apperception Test – Human (CAT-H) – ages 3–10 • Roberts Apperception Test – ages 6–15 • Thematic Apperception Test (TAT) – ages 7–18 • Rorschach – ages 5–18 • HTP

	• Begin asking questions about sex (6–9 years) • Interest in games related to sexuality • Friendships are situation-specific • Understands right/wrong • Understands that rules guide behavior/play and provide structure • Social roles are inflexible • Less fantasy play, more focus on sports and board games	• DAP • KFD • Sentence Completion Tests (SCT) • BASC-3 • ASEBA • Millon Preadolescent Clinical Inventory (M-PACI) – ages 9–12
Adolescence (12–14)	• Self-conscious about physical appearance (early or late development) • Body image is subjective • Emotionally labile • Increased ability to consider various solutions/ strategies to deal with stress • Able to distinguish genuine emotion with friends from managed emotional displays with others • Seeks activities for intense emotional experience • Risky behavior • Rejects parental standards, psychological distance • Focuses on peer group for support and identity • Social acceptance relies on conformity to observable traits/roles • Ambivalence about sexual relationships	• Rorschach • Roberts • TAT • HTP • DAP • KFD • SCT • BASC-3 • ASEBA • Millon Adolescent Clinical Inventory (MACI) – ages 13–18
Adolescence (15 17)	• Increased consideration of others' values/beliefs • Increased awareness of own emotional cycles enables insightful coping • Identity organized around attitudes, behaviors and values to construct a more coherent whole • Identity integrates cognitive and emotional components toward a more positive self-image • Friendships based on understanding, trust and loyalty • Self-revelation is first step toward intimacy • Conscious choice about which adults to trust • Respects honesty from adults • May become sexually active	• Rorschach • TAT • HTP • DAP • KFD • SCT • BASC-3 • ASEBA • MACI • Minnesota Multiphasic Personality Inventory – Adolescent (MMPI-A) – ages 14–18

Sources: Rycus & Hughes (1998); and Saarni (2000).

Developing Accommodations and Interventions

Once the extent of a child's externalizing and internalizing symptoms have been identified through observation and assessment, accommodations can be put in place and interventions can be made. It is important to note that, often, externalizing and internalizing symptoms are co-morbid (Willner et al., 2016). The following sections indicate specific interventions. It is important to individualize each accommodation or intervention. Academic support may also be warranted. Furthermore, it is important to remember that all of the following accommodations and strategies are best implemented within the context of a holding environment (Winnicott, 1965) that has a foundation based in the relationship formed between the teacher or specialist and the child.

Please note that the following accommodations are not divided into two categories regarding which would work best for internalizing symptoms or externalizing symptoms. This is intentional and due to the fact that often, the same accommodation can support a child with either or both types of symptoms. *How* the accommodation is implemented and individualized for each student is important to meet their unique presentation.

General Academic Accommodations and Strategies

- Preview schedule, tasks and content.
- Set clear and consistent expectations, consequences, and routines.
- Use checklists.
- Use self-monitoring checklist.
- Provide time to process emotional upset (with use of visuals and decreased language).
- Allow access to quiet space or separate work area.
- Implement positive intervention plan.
- Designate an identified adult for support.
- Maintain consistency across environments.
- Build relationships with adults.
- Allow access to therapeutic staff members as needed.
- Provide support during transitions.
- Provide social skills support.
- Use individualized social stories.
- Allow access to emotional tools that promote self-regulation (feelings thermometer, scale from 1–5, etc.).
- Use a behavior or emotions (mood) chart.
- Adults should “adapt and roll” with emotional resistance and tendency to shut down.
- Individual begins the day in the resource center, checks in and previews daily schedule.
- Modify workload.
- Allow extra time on assignments and tests.
- Ask student to restate directions before beginning a task/assignment.
- Provide extra time for student to formulate thoughts before responding.
- Establish preferential seating.
- Break down assignments into small manageable chunks.
- Allow opportunities for movement breaks.
- Implement social problem-solving.
- Preview new situations and environments (using visuals).
- Provide individual counseling.
- Engage in social skills group.
- Adults attune to student’s emotional state and maintain awareness of “triggers.”
- Explicitly and frequently teach social rules and skills.
- Model appropriate responses to social situations.
- Engage student in role-play opportunities.

- Explain rules/rationales behind social exchanges.
- Target perspective-taking skills.
- Teach student to accurately label his/her emotions.
- Teach student to accurately label the emotional status of others (based on facial cues, verbal cues, etc.).
- Provide opportunities for student to contribute to classroom environment or assume responsibility (hand out worksheets, etc.).
- Specify rewards for following the rules and consequences for disobeying rules.
- Model responses to potential triggers for escalation.
- Teach student to describe a conflict or problem, identify possible responses, and evaluate response.
- Immediately praise appropriate behavior.
- Engage in regular and consistent communication between family members, counselors, and community-based service providers.
- Modify/accommodate work demands based upon the student's performance levels/stamina.
- Assign classmate as volunteer assistant.
- Allow food or beverages in class (or have access to them).
- Make syllabus and textbooks available early.
- Offer private feedback on academic performance.
- Provide advance notice of assignments.
- Allow handwritten rather than typed assignments.
- Allow written assignments in lieu of oral presentations (and vice versa).
- Provide access to a well-lit or brightly lit environment.
- Provide extra books for home.
- Planned ignoring for selected behaviors that are in need of decreasing.
- Offer choices within limits.
- Reflect and process after behavioral incidents.
- Make a plan with the student to decrease inappropriate behaviors and develop appropriate behaviors.
- Engage in frequent and consistent communication between home and school.
- Engage in frequent and consistent communication between all team members.

Based on: College Committee for Disability Issues (2008); Reinstein & Burau (2014); and Crundwell & Killu (2007).

Addressing Social/Emotional Functioning

In previous chapters, this section has broken the functional domain into groups based on how the domain is assessed, potential accommodations and intervention, and how interventions are implemented. In this chapter, a different approach is taken. Our emotions have the ability to impact every aspect of functioning, including both social and academic. To address this, the following sections outline how to develop therapeutic relationships with individual students who are struggling with internalizing and externalizing symptoms. Difficult classroom behaviors will also be addressed. This therapeutic relationship becomes the conduit through which all instruction takes place. As research indicates, it has the potential to be a healing and life-altering experience for our students.

Cultivating a Relationship

It has been demonstrated that the relationship between students and teachers can have an impact on the social/emotional development of a student as well as impact his or her academic performance (Sobol & Pianta, 2012). High-quality relationships with teachers appear to decelerate the deleterious effects of risk and promote healthy functioning for children with internalizing and externalizing problems (Baker, 2006; Baker et al., 2008; Ladd & Burgess, 2001; Silver et al., 2005). For children with externalizing problems, perceptions of teacher relationships that are perceived as close are associated with improved social skills (Berry & O'Connor, 2010), peer relations (Gazelle, 2006), and academic outcomes (Baker, 2006). Students who exhibit externalizing problems also benefit from warm and supportive relationships with teachers (Hamre & Pianta, 2001; Meehan et al., 2003). Positive relationships with students who exhibit externalizing behaviors are associated with higher reading skills (Baker et al., 2008), the deceleration of externalizing behaviors (Silver et al., 2005), and higher academic performance (Baker, 2006) compared to similar children who do not have the opportunity to engage in positive relationships.

The potential positive impact of the teacher–student relationship can be explained through the lens of attachment theory and research. While most research in this area has focused on parent–child relationships, teacher–student relationships can provide the opportunity for a child to participate in a warm and caring relationship outside of the home. Similar to parents, teachers have the opportunity to provide a secure base and safe haven for students. Teachers are also in a position to provide affective feedback to students and to observe the effect of the student and either mirror it, explain it, or provide an alternative (Verschueren, 2015).

Research indicates that an important aspect of the teacher–student relationship is the teacher's ability to be sensitive to the needs of the child (Bakermans-Kranenburg et al., 2003). High teacher sensitivity toward vulnerable students serves as a protective factor (Buyse et al., 2008). Regarding attachment, teacher sensitivity toward a student indicates the teacher is highly observational and in tune with a child's behavior. Attachment theory addresses the concept of attachment behaviors, which relate to the types of behaviors (e.g., crying, calling, babbling, smiling, clinging, and crawling toward) in which infants engage in order to maintain proximity to caregivers and get basic needs met (Bowlby, 1988). As an individual grows, the child engages in more developmentally sophisticated attachment behaviors, including non-verbal and verbal means for maintaining proximity. Teachers are in a position to carefully observe a child's behavior through this lens, aided by an understanding of the child's neuropsychological strengths and vulnerabilities, and respond to the child in order to meet their needs.

Before attachment theory was clearly defined, Donald Winnicott (1965) developed the concept of the *good enough mother* (or parent/caregiver). This concept attempts to address the impossible task of *always* being able to attune to the child and develop the perfect relational space. After all, parents are human and have their own feelings and reactions. Likewise, teachers can be the "good enough teacher."

Attempt to closely observe the child, learn their subtle and not-so-subtle cues, and provide intervention or affective feedback. Winnicott also coined the term ***the holding environment***, which refers to the relational space between a mother (or parent/guardian) and child. Within this literal and metaphorical space, the child's needs are met. This includes soothing the child, providing safety and protection, being aware of the child's sensory needs, providing structure and routine, and being carefully attuned to be aware of when to respond with flexibility to a child's behavior in order to meet the changing demands of development. As the child matures, the hope is that they will internalize the "holding" provided through the relationship, and be able to care for themselves as they grow increasingly independent. Outside of the parent–child dyad, the concept of the holding environment can be applied to the teacher–student relationship and even to the physical space of the classroom setting (Reinstein, 2006). How to do so will be thoroughly discussed in Chapter 7.

Using this theoretical orientation, combined with the results of neuropsychological and psychological evaluations, teachers and specialists can make careful observation, as a "good enough" teacher would. Through this observation, they develop insight into how a student's behavior might actually be a form of attachment behavior (Bowlby, 1988) indicating a need that is not being met, the inability to self-soothe, or the desire for a protective and secure relationship. Then, applying evaluation results, a Child–World System (Holmes-Bernstein & Weiler, 2000) can be constructed. In doing so, areas of "match" or "mismatch" between the child's needs and demands of the school setting can be better understood. In the case of mismatches, supports can be modified to create a better match, essentially building a holding environment for the student.

Relationships Have Two Sides: Know Thyself

The concepts presented above of sensitivity, attunement, provision of intervention, and affective feedback, and even the good enough mother (or teacher) and the holding environment can create a vision of a loving and well-regulated classroom. However, school environments are often busy with quick transitions and too little time for important conversations. These students can be frustrating, difficult to connect with, and appear lazy and unmotivated. As a result, teachers can feel overworked, tired, stressed, and frustrated. Is this, then, what is brought from the teacher into the teacher–student relationship? How can you tell when you are truly bringing your best version of yourself into the classroom and how do you forgive yourself when you do not?

Beyond how the demands of the school environment may impact a teacher's mood or state of mind is the way in which a student impacts a teacher's mood or state of mind. In what ways do you think about a child or respond to them? Have you ever wondered if a child would be better off living with you rather than with their parent(s)? Have you ever been so frustrated with the behavior of a student that you wanted to yell and scream? What is it about that child, and not another child, that elicits this primal reaction? Are there some students for whom you have endless patience and others who immediately push your buttons? When discussing students with other teachers, do they have the same reactions or widely different feelings from you about the same student? When a student skips class or doesn't turn in assignments on time, does it feel like a personal slight? Do you relate to students of a similar cultural background better than those from different backgrounds? These reactions to students are common. They can be confusing and they may impact the way in which teachers relate to students, grade their work, or design and implement interventions.

Contemporary psychodynamic theory states the importance of paying attention to and understanding why some people elicit emotional reactions within us (Hyman, 2012). This is contradictory to some current notions that teachers are expected to leave their emotions outside of the classroom despite the impossibility of doing so (Britzman, 2009; Britzman & Dippo, 2000). A different approach involves investigating and examining the feelings to ensure that they are not driving an intervention, but rather that a true perception of how to meet the student's needs is driving the intervention. For a teacher, the task at hand might be to learn how to tolerate emotional outbursts, non-compliance, opposition, late work, or disruption of a calm classroom environment or learning of others in order to maintain a facilitating relationship and environment that provides the student with the emotional and educational context needed for growth (Min Shim, 2014). This allows the teacher to set limits not out of frustration, but because the child needs boundaries in order to grow. Teachers must undergo self-examination to understand *why* these behaviors are more or less frustrating in different students. Are the behaviors frustrating because they challenge your culture of origin (for example, timely arrival is a cultural norm), they remind you of how a person from another relationship behaved, you grew up in poverty and the student has resources they are not taking advantage of or are grateful for . . . etc., etc., etc.? Expectations teachers have for their students and their behavior often arise out of their own experiences and training. Bringing these expectations into the relational space must be done thoughtfully so that, as a teacher, you understand what you are bringing into the relationship, how this promotes or inhibits your observations of a student, and what intervention direction should be taken.

The Value of Play

Thus far, we have established that in order to treat social/emotional issues such as internalizing and externalizing problems, the attachment relationship between the student and teacher is paramount (Geddes, 2006; Elkind, 2007). Building and maintaining this relationship requires that teachers have a strong understanding of themselves and how their perceptions and experiences impact the relationship. Aside from being caring and sensitive to a child's needs, how do you cultivate this relationship?

Play is an essential tool for teachers to develop relationships with students. Play can be done with an individual or within a group context. Winnicott recognized the link between play and attachment while observing mothers playing peek-a-boo with their children. The close proximity and careful watching of the child's reaction to various faces and noises creates a relational space (1974). Beyond infancy, play can be used with children, teens, and young adults with attachment needs as a vehicle for repairing damaged attachment (Jennings, 2011). Play is about connection (Rogers, 2011). Engaging in playful activities can be the means for developing and sustaining a variety of relationships as well as for exploring, learning, and developing empathy (Elkind, 2007; Szalavitz and Perry, 2011).

Defining play can be difficult because it is culturally bound, highly individualized, and takes many forms. It can be highly physical, rough-and-tumble, or just the joy of running. Play can involve pretending and imagination, such as using a banana as a phone or a napkin as a hat. Engaging in fantasy play allows individuals to explore the differences between reality and fantasy. Narrative play involves the creation of storylines and can help individuals better understand their life experiences (Brown & Vaughn, 2009). Play can involve building, constructing, and creating new objects from various materials. Structured play takes the form of sports or games with rules and limits, and is less open-ended and potentially more containing (Landreth, 2002).

In addition to the various types of play, it is important to keep in mind its developmental trajectory. Play looks very different at different ages and stages. Thus, how you engage an individual through play should match their developmental stage. Sometimes, different stages can occur during the same developmental period. The following information is based on Mildred Parten's stages of play (1932).

- Unoccupied Play (0–2 years old): the child is engaged in moving their body somewhat randomly or attending to objects that are near to them. Due to their nascent stages of development, adults and other people primarily engage the child.
- Solitary Play (2–3 years old): the child has intentional movements and engages with toys. Children learn how to entertain or engage themselves.
- Onlooker Play (2:6–3:6 years old and other ages): the child intently observes the action and play of others, but does not have the skills to engage in the activity. They may point or ask questions and intentionally engage others.
- Parallel Play (2:6–3:6 and other ages): children play with the same toys, in proximity of each other, but are not directly engaged with each other. They may observe each other.
- Associative Play (3–4 years old and other ages): children directly engage each other, but may not be focused on a common goal. They talk with each other, trade play items, and develop play scripts, but the scripts may differ from one another. Cooperation and problem-solving begin to develop. Learning how to share occurs.
- Cooperative Play (begins in ages 4–6 and lasts until latency): children become fully engaged with each other and share common goals, and self-made rules often develop. Teamwork and cooperation are observable. Often, a leader or two emerges within the group.
- Latency and teen years: play begins to shift from imaginative narrative play to a more hobbies-based activity. As the child matures, their interests shift. They move from playing Legos on the floor to discussing their favorite music. They develop specific interests and hobbies.

Understanding and observing the stages of play allows adults to engage children at their developmental level. During latency and into the early teen years, this can be difficult as the child sheds their younger means for play and becomes more mature, vacillating between the two stages.

In addition to creating a venue for connection in relationship, play creates connections between neurons, neurological systems, and different parts of the brain (Brown &

Vaughn, 2009), linking thought, emotion, reasoning, and creative centers. In preschool-aged children, recent research indicates correlations between engaging in fantasy play and the development of executive functions including working memory, self-regulation, inhibitory control, and shifting attention (Thibodeau et al., 2016; S. M. Carlson et al., 2014; Pierucci et al., 2014). This supports the notion that play promotes self-regulation and the ability to navigate reality and fantasy (Vygotsky, 1978). As the play develops, objects become representational (such as the napkin hat), and abstract thought and the use of symbols becomes important (Woolley & Tullos, 2008).

In addition to the development of executive functions and abstract thought, research demonstrates that playful activities can have a direct influence on the development of specific academic skills. This is true for both unstructured play and teacher-guided play (Johnson et al., 2005). For example, construction activities such as building with blocks or playing with Legos correlate with the development of math skills. In teens, structural building activities correlate with mathematical performance (Casey et al., 2012). In 3- to 4-year-olds, using instructions to build a model correlates with early math skills (Verdine et al., 2013). Other research suggests that construction play in preschool can have long-term effects on logic-mathematical knowledge (Stannard et al., 2001). Spatial ability, required for construction play, has been linked to scientific reasoning when taking verbal and non-verbal intelligence into account (Mayer et al., 2014).

In relation to literacy development, children engaged in pretend play are likely to talk more, which is associated with a larger vocabulary and more advanced oral language skills. This association is linked to literacy development (Han et al., 2010). Recent studies on the effects of socio-dramatic play on the development of narrative reading skills, or the ability to understand and retell what has been heard, indicate that pretend play can have a positive impact. While more research is required to validate these findings, several studies indicate this correlation (Nicolopoulou & Ilgaz, 2013). In making use of guided play in the classroom, teachers should take on various roles including onlooker, co-player, and, sometimes, play leader (Roskos et al., 2004).

How Games Promote Pro-Social Behavior

It can be argued that most games promote pro-social behavior, regardless of the game. For example, board games teach children to take turns, wait their turn, tolerate setbacks, tolerate losing, and learn how to win, and provide time spent with others around a common interest. Children displaying externalizing symptoms may need extra support during game times to develop these skills. Therapeutic behavior plans can be developed to promote pro-social behavior (such as waiting one's turn) or provide clear consequences for breaking social norms (calling another child names or intentionally destroying the game board when faced with a challenge). Perhaps most importantly, if issues arise during game-play, space can be made to help the child learn why they have the feelings and behaviors they do in reaction to losing (such as poor self-esteem due to learning disabilities (LD) or trauma history) and develop coping strategies that will allow them to foster social relationships (such as scripts for how to appropriately state disappointment at a loss or taking a break to re-regulate themselves).

Some researchers are investigating the effect of combining Cognitive Behavior Therapy (CBT) with game-based activities. Combining game-based play with CBT can be used as a therapeutic modality for working with children who have experienced sexual abuse. Participants in research studies have demonstrated improvements with both internalizing and externalizing behavior problems. This may be in part because the participants remained engaged in the therapeutic activity and had a lower attrition rate than those involved in other therapeutic interventions (Misurell et al., 2014).

When using games to develop social skills, be sure to find games that utilize the cognitive strengths of the child rather than their difficulties. If a child struggles with verbal reasoning and you invite them to play Scrabble, and the intent of the game time is to build social skills, you are now asking the child to work on *two* of their challenges, which is harder work and may lead to more frustration. Instead, choose a game that plays to their strengths. If they have strong perceptual reasoning skills, find a game that utilizes that skill. As a result, their self-esteem will increase, they will have a positive experience, and they will potentially be more motivated to work through the social and emotional difficulties. If the student is older, be sure to find games that match their cognitive skill set but are not infantilizing.

Therapeutic Language and the Use of Metaphor

Part of developing a relationship, engaging in play, and recognizing and addressing internalizing or externalizing symptoms is *how* we speak *to* and *with* a child. For example, a 12-year-old who is diagnosed with profound dyslexia but has a verbal comprehension of 110 should not be spoken to as a young child because they read at a first-grade level. Instead, they should be spoken to at an age and skill level commensurate with their abilities. Conversely, a 12-year-old who struggles with verbal comprehension may need adults to speak to and with them in more simple concrete language, avoiding the use of confusing metaphors and abstract concepts (unless the metaphors and concepts have been previewed with the child).

In either scenario, it is possible to develop specific terms, phrases, jokes, and metaphors within the relationship that address the individual's challenging emotions and/or behaviors. Metaphors develop in the context of the relationship and careful observation. In this way, the child (or their parent) shares their own experiences and understanding of their strengths and vulnerabilities. This observation is not limited to verbal exchanges only, but can also include gestures, play, level of kinetic energy, use of music, movement, or visual arts. Through this observation, the adult can engage the individual in her own space and metaphor, make sense of it, reflect, and respond, and share their own experience when appropriate. A common language arises out of these experiences, fostering the development and maintenance of the holding environment (Reinstein, 2006). The development and use of therapeutic language and metaphor is not restricted to individuals but can also become part of a group culture.

For example, a student referred to as Sally exhibited manic-like symptoms through long monologues spoken at a very rapid rate, a rate so fast most listeners were lost in gibberish. Interrupting the monologue resulted in great frustration for Sally. She would also begin to rock or bounce in her seat and her gestures would become erratic. After a few weeks of this, the teacher asked Sally, "What does it feel like to talk for so long and so fast?" Sally responded with, "I can't describe it. Can I draw it?" At this point, Sally took out papers and markers and drew a tsunami engulfing a small figure. The teacher and Sally discussed the wave and the possibility of building a dam or channels to help guide the flow of water. In this way, the behavior was discussed, but not in accusatory or degrading means. Subsequently, whenever Sally began a monologue the teacher made a gesture indicating an approaching wave. Sally would stop the monologue, engage in a strategy to slow herself down, and relay the information in a way that others could be receptive. In time, Sally and the teacher identified that the waves were the strongest when Sally was feeling anxious.

In addition to the use of individualized metaphors, students can benefit from a common language that is used to describe and discuss emotions and behaviors. This common language can be shared across classrooms and environments (home and school, for example) in order to simplify the student's experience of therapeutic language. The Community Therapeutic Day School has developed a glossary of terms used in all classrooms, creating continuity which contributes to the holding environment. This language is then shared with the parents, particularity language that is effective with their child and which can be utilized in the home. Often parents, rightfully overwhelmed by their child's behavior, are at a loss for words, unable to talk to their child or discuss difficult situations. This glossary of terms provides holding for the parents as well. For example, disruptive or dangerous behavior can be the result of the child's difficulty managing overwhelming feelings. These feelings can be mad, sad, excited, etc. These overwhelming feelings are referred to as "big feelings" in all classrooms. This term is used to help the student identify the root of their behavior and develop individualized management strategies.

Therapeutic Behavior Plans

Both internalizing and externalizing problems can be expressed through behavioral difficulties. Aggressive behavior, rude behavior, truancy, incomplete homework, checking out in class, shutting down, etc., can be part of the behavioral presentation. Beginning in 1997 and again in 2004 with the reauthorization of the Individuals with Disabilities Education Improvement Act (IDEIA), educators have been required to develop and implement behavior intervention plans (BIPs). These plans are intended to identify the relationship between behavior problems and student learning and then ameliorate the problem behavior. A BIP is intended to define a specific targeted behavior that needs to be altered. When the student either engages in the desired behavior or does not engage in the undesired behavior, they are rewarded (or receive a consequence). The hope is that the undesired behavior ceases and the more pro-social behavior generalizes to all environments.

While BIPs have become a mandated element of special education, improperly developing and implementing behavior plans can be harmful to students. Without a clear understanding of the underlying causes for the disruptive behavior, not only will the plans be ineffective but, even more damaging, the student will experience more failure, missed opportunities to get needs met, and inadequate relationships. The lens of the relationship and how it can facilitate the development and implementation of BIPs is essential. Without the essential relational component, the plan is merely addressing the behavior, and not the needs of the whole child. In order to develop a thoughtful BIP that can be used therapeutically as part of the holding environment, several factors must be considered:

- The student must be carefully observed. During this observation, there must be consensus on the unfavorable behavior. There should be clear measurement of the frequency of the behavior. Antecedents and consequences of the targeted behavior should be identified as well as identification of potential reinforcers (Killu, 2008).
- Don't stop collecting information while observing direct antecedents! Consider what are referred to as *setting events*, or occurrences outside of the moment that may impact the student's behavior or the effectiveness of the BIP. A poor night's sleep, an argument with a parent or peer, illness, etc., can have an impact on the student's behavior (Jolivette et al., 1999).
- BIPs operate on the premise that a reward is the outcome of desired behavior or a negative reinforcement is the result of undesired behavior, with an outcome of either promoting or extinguishing specific behaviors. However, if the frequency of the target behavior is not changing, the reinforcement is not working. Careful observation of the student during the plan must occur. If the plan is not working, one must consider that secondary reinforcers (such as getting attention, even if it is for "getting into trouble") are somehow reinforcing the undesired behavior (Maag, 2001; Cooper et al., 2007).
- The plan must be implemented accurately and consistently. The plan must also be efficient, appropriate to the situation and context and, most of all, understood by the student and those who are utilizing it (Killu, 2008). If the plan is not accepted by those who implement it or benefit from it, it will likely fail.
- Bear in mind that many inappropriate behaviors are the result of vulnerability in emotional, cognitive or other types of functioning. Without understanding the underlying vulnerability, the plan will not address the entirety of the issue at hand. The plan must not only attempt to eliminate the undesired behavior but also focus on remediating or supporting the vulnerability (Killu, 2008).
- The desired behavior will hopefully maintain and generalize to other environments once the plan ceases. Students may need to be taught self-monitoring and self-management strategies in order to achieve these goals (Todd et al., 1997).
- Rather than simply focusing on behavior change, promote student growth and achievement by facilitating their understanding of their own behavior and emotional experience (Crone & Horner, 2003; Sugai & Horner, 2006). This entails having conversations with the student, developing goals together, developing self-understanding, and supporting their perceived failures and successes. It is necessary to individualize the BIP to the student, situation, teacher, and family circumstances.

Another element that can be included in behavior plans or behavior management is the use of time-out. The use of time-out has been effective in reducing a variety of behaviors including tantrums, inappropriate social behavior, yelling, aggression, time spent out-of-seat, and inappropriate verbalizations (Alberto et al., 2002; Mortimer et al., 1998).

Literature indicates a variety of types and ways of using time-out, but for our purposes in this manual "time-out" refers to ***contingent observation***. This occurs when the student is in the classroom, seated separately from the group activity and watching from the periphery for a period of time (Wolf et al., 2006).

Time-outs of this nature should be used thoughtfully, ethically, and carefully. The previously identified considerations for BIPs should be made when considering the use of time-out. Some advocate that time-out can be used to help children learn how to self-regulate (Mercier, 2014). In Winnicottian terms, time-out can be used as part of the holding environment. Students are unable to regulate themselves, so an external resource (the teacher) helps the child regulate through their tone, observation, and limits. The intent is that, with the help of the teacher, the student will learn their own cues that lead to difficult moments, internalize the support, learn to stop themselves, and utilize pro-social behavior to meet their needs (Reinstein, 2006). In order for time-outs to be effective, one must:

- Integrate other methods of behavior change. Reinforce positive behavior with praise and reward, have conversations with the student to develop awareness and alternate strategies for their difficult behaviors, advocate for their needs, and provide pro-social coping strategies.
- Build a positive relationship with the student and show positive regard throughout your time together (Wolf et al., 2006).
- When a student is sent to time-out, use a calm and clear tone of voice. Use time-out before personal frustration occludes your own thought process and judgment (Mercier, 2014).
- Carefully choose the location of the time-out area. It could be the student's desk with all materials removed. It could be a chair in a somewhat separate space (Wolf et al., 2006). Some advocate that the space should be free of toys or activities, while others assert that tools be made available to help the child calm down (Mercier, 2014). The space should be well-lit, well-ventilated, and observable by adults.
- Preview the concept of time-out with the student (and their parents). Identify with the student behaviors that result in time-out. Preview the location and expected behaviors in time-out. Have an idea for the duration of time used in time-out.
- Observe the child to ascertain the time-out is not accidentally reinforcing unwanted behaviors, such as avoiding work.
- Train all staff members who will interact with the student regarding the time-out plan.
- When a time-out is complete, ***debrief*** the experience with the student (Colvin, 1993, 1997). During this conversation, the student and teacher identify the behavior that resulted in time-out and replacement behaviors that are better options. This conversation should convey care, respect, and concern. The relationship between the student and teacher can also be discussed in order to ameliorate any lingering negative emotions. Debriefing should occur when the student is ready and able to rejoin the group and stay on task.

- As with BIPs, be aware that the inappropriate behaviors are the result of an unmet need, neuropsychological vulnerability, or psychiatric condition. Provide opportunity for the student to get their need met appropriately or provide alternative options to address the vulnerability or psychiatric condition.

There has been debate over the effectiveness, usefulness, and ethical consideration of using time-out for behavior management. As noted above, studies indicate its usefulness. Misuse of time-out occurs when educators don't understand the purpose of time-out or overuse it (Lang, 1997). Proper use of time-out requires the teacher to be aware of their attitude toward the student and be sure that they are not using time-out for their own gain (such as 10 minutes of quiet) but rather for the best interest of the student (Wolf et al., 2006). The intent of time-out is not to establish control over the child, cause embarrassment or shame, or socially alienate the child, but to teach awareness and self-control.

Internalizing and Externalizing Symptoms in School

As we have discussed, our emotional states can impact various areas of functioning. The following section briefly presents some research indicating how internalizing and externalizing symptoms can impact functioning in the school environment. This material is presented to highlight the importance of utilizing a therapeutic approach.

- Regarding social and emotional development, childhood peer rejection predicts externalizing behaviors during the school-age years (Hymel et al., 1990) and into adolescence (Coie et al., 1995). Studies indicate a relationship between internalizing behaviors/symptoms and social skills that is similar to the chicken and egg scenario. For example, social difficulties and isolation in second grade are linked to internalizing behaviors three years later (Hymel et al., 1990) and increased social isolation is associated with depressed mood in boys aged 12 to 15 (Larson et al., 1990). This suggests that social difficulties lead to internalizing behaviors and symptoms. However, symptoms of anxiety and depression have predictive significance for several emotional disorders and show linkages with poor peer social adjustment (Rubin et al., 2006; Harrington & Clark, 1998).
- It is documented that children and adolescents with LD have difficulties with school adjustment and experience increased internalizing problems (Greenham, 1999; Huntington & Bender, 1993; Maag & Reid, 2006). Studies also show that these internalizing problems persist into adulthood (Klassen et al., 2013). The type of LD may impact the individual's internalizing symptoms and longevity as well as other factors (Grafen et al., 2015). It has been noted that reading problems elevate a child's odds of engaging in problem behaviors, even when studies are designed to control for other factors such as poor attention and SES- and demographic-related confounds. Poor reading ability in first grade constantly acts as a predictor for problem behavior in third grade. In attempting to understand causation for this issue,

Morgan et al. (2008) contend there are four potential pathways for risk: (a) early reading problems strongly predict later reading problems; (b) early behavior problems predict reading problems; (c) early reading problems modestly-to-moderately predict a general set of behavior problems; and (d) one type of early behavior problem that relates to self-regulation strongly predicts later reading problems.

- While there are few studies that investigate the relationship between math skills and externalizing symptoms, the few that have been done make some connection between math disabilities and diagnoses that encompass externalizing symptoms. For example, children in second and third grade who have difficulties in math tend to exhibit higher levels of attention problems and concurrent social difficulties. Children learning at the lowest end of math achievement are more likely to develop or display symptoms related to ADHD, social problems, and potentially conduct disorder or oppositional defiant disorder (Wu et al., 2014).

Chapter 6 Appendix: Social/Emotional Functioning Interventions

USING ART TO RECOGNIZE FEELINGS

Goal: Develop awareness of feelings/emotions over the course of a day and how they are experienced in the body. This facilitates self-awareness and can lead to the development of appropriate coping skills.

Materials: Body Outline worksheet; markers, crayons, or colorful pens. Use of a feelings face chart may be helpful.

Directions: Before handing out the Body Outline worksheet, ask the classroom (or individual) to think about different feelings or emotions they have felt throughout the day. Differentiate between feelings (tired, hungry, cold, etc.) and emotions (sad, happy, mad, etc.). Ask them to imagine that each sensation is a color. Hand out the Body Outline worksheet. Have them write down the feeling or emotion on the line on the right side of the page. Instruct them to color the box in with the color (or pattern) that matches the sensation. Once they have finished this step, ask them to imagine where in their body they feel the sensation. Ask them to decorate the outlined body with the colors. If they feel it is appropriate to go outside of the body outline, let them know this is okay. Once they have all finished coloring their outlines, ask them to share if they are comfortable.

Adaptations:

- If the child has graphomotor issues, offer to scribe their feelings.
- Use a facial feelings chart to help the student identify potential feelings.
- If they are resistant and don't write down feelings or emotions but rather provide colors, go with it! Accept what they do and don't struggle over it. It is their expression of their experience.
- This activity could be used with an individual when they are escalating to provide a non-verbal means of expression. It is best if they have prior exposure to the activity when used this way.
- This activity can be used in a group as a check-in as a way to establish how each group member is doing on a daily basis.

Based on: Gil (2006).

Body Outline

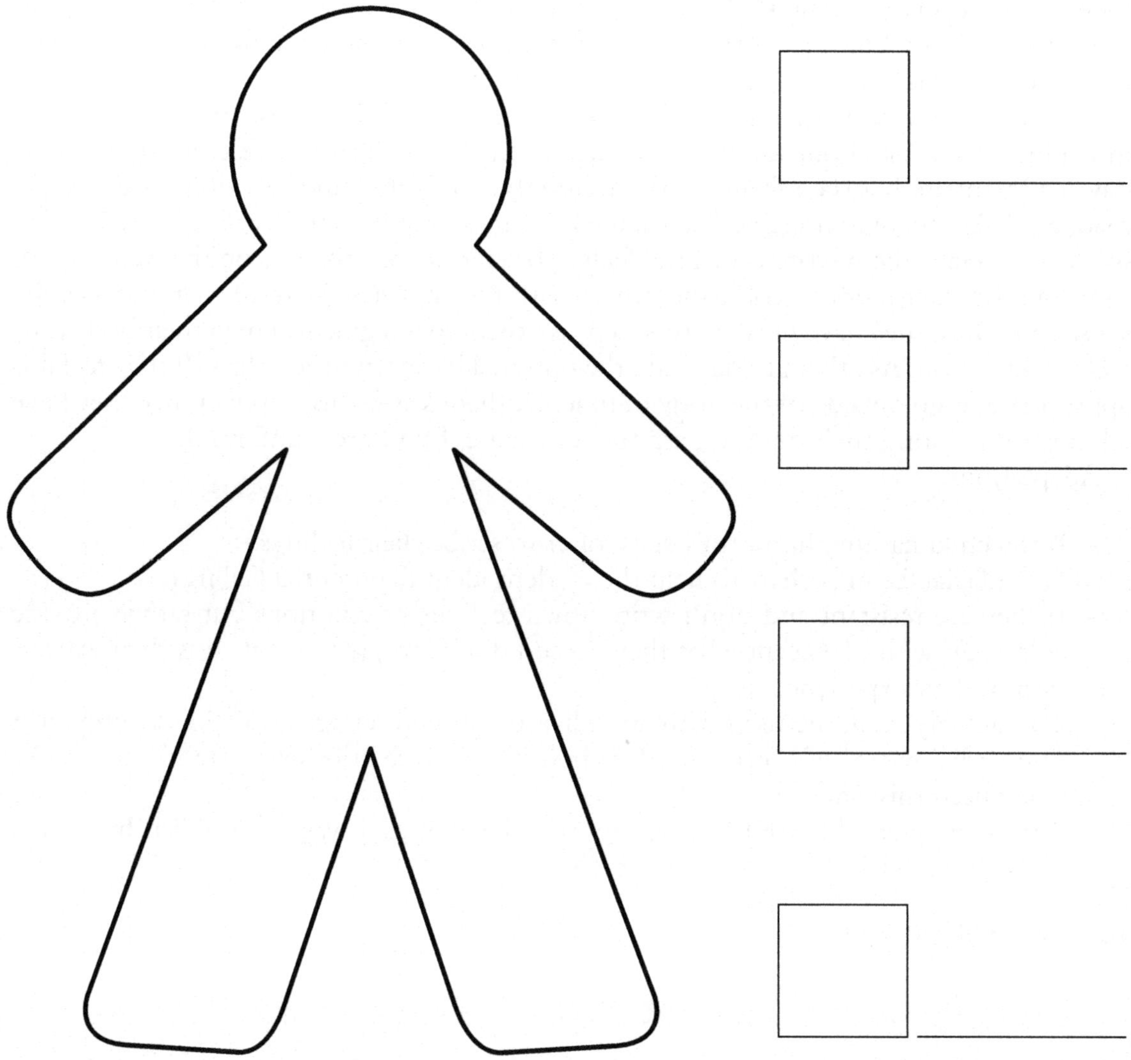

EXAMPLE OF PLAY INTERVENTION FOR INTERNALIZING PROBLEMS

Goal: Provide a format/space for apprehensive children to find a voice and share their thoughts through the use of a puppet.

Materials: Use puppets that are already made, or make your own. This can be done using socks, glue, fabric and yarn, or paper lunch bags, glue paper, stickers, etc.

Directions: Ask the child (children) to make a puppet and guide them through the process. Once the puppet is made, interview it. Ask the puppet what they would do to solve certain problems (such as some of the problems the child is currently facing).

Adaptation: This project can be age-sensitive. Make sure the individual won't feel infantilized by the activity.

Based on: Carolyn J. Narcavage in Kaduson & Schaefer (1997).

EXAMPLE OF PLAY INTERVENTION FOR EXTERNALIZING PROBLEMS

Goal: Develop an understanding of what causes different individuals to feel angry, that everyone can feel angry, and that we can learn appropriate means for managing angry feelings.

Materials: Pile of different types of blocks (equal amounts for each person).

Directions: The group (or teacher–student pair) will make a group sculpture. In order to add a block to the group sculpture, you share an event that can make you angry. The adult starts with something simple like "sitting in traffic" and adds a block. Everyone takes turns adding to the tower. Once the tower is completed, an individual is asked to make a "mad face" and knock the block tower down.

Adaptations:

- Post-It notes with the events that lead to mad feelings can be written and then posted to the blocks in order to help track what has been said.
- This could be used for other feelings as well.

Based on: a game by Patricia Davidson as cited in Kaduson & Schaefer (1997).

EXAMPLE OF USING PLAY IN A READING LESSON

Goal: Facilitate learning of early reading skills through playful activities.

- Fish Me Up: Children use magnetic fishing rods to "fish" magnetic flash cards. Each card has a letter, syllable, sentence phrase, etc., depending on reading level. The child fishes up two cards that match. They then read the cards to combine the letters. Doing this intentionally to make real words and sentences and also gibberish can help develop skills.
- Putting on Socks: The teacher (or students) writes letters on socks. The children put the socks on and then line up, putting their feet together to spell words. They can decide on the words or use a grade-level appropriate spelling list.
- Bowling of Letters: Using empty plastic bottles, the teacher writes syllables or letters on them with a marker. The teacher (or a peer) organizes the bottles several feet away from the child. The student then rolls the ball, knocks over a "pin," and identifies what is written on the bottle.

Adaptation: Make sure playful activities match both the reading skill level and the developmental level of the child.

Based on: Ali et al. (2011).

EXAMPLE OF USING PLAY IN A MATH LESSON

Goal: Facilitate various mathematical skills through play.

- Block Play: During free play, allow the students access to various types of blocks. For more structured play, provide blocks and ask children to build various structures with them. Ask the children to build specific features (such as doors, windows or rooms). This promotes early geometric and spatial skills (Kamii et al., 2004).
- Ping-Pong Math Toss: Using paper cups, write single-digit numbers on the bottom of cups counting up from 0 to 9. Arrange cups in a shoe box or other easily transportable box. Using ping-pong balls, have the students toss a ball into the cups. When they get two numbers (such as 5 and 2), have them perform a math operation on the numbers (adding, subtracting, or multiplying). For dividing, you must have the large numbers with their dividends. Students can make their own boxes to promote motivation. You can have them toss the ball several times to practice adding (or other operations) with a larger numbers sentence. If students do this in pairs, they can take turns tossing the ball and writing the number sentences.
- Play various dice games such as Farkle and Yahtzee. These games engage working memory and can also be used to discuss probability and ratios.
- Play games that promote math skills. For example, Battleship helps students understand the use of an X and Y axis. Mastermind helps children learn about patterns and algebraic thinking. Various card games promote numeracy skills and engage working memory.
- Combine literature and math activities. For example, read *Caps for Sale* (Slobodkina, 1947) to discuss the value of the hats and money. Use the different colors of hats to create groups and patterns.

THERAPEUTIC LANGUAGE GLOSSARY

"Acting inappropriately": to act or speak in a manner inconsistent with rules of safety or rules of respect for self and others.

"Be safe": a reminder to behave in a safe manner. May refer to actions or language that could lead to someone being hurt.

"Be the boss of yourself": a verbal reminder to stay in control and behave in a safe manner. An attempt to reinforce a child's desire to master self-control and independence while reassuring them of their connection with the adult.

"Goofy": acting in a silly way that may or may not become inappropriate (you can also develop your own term for this that is shared between you and the child).

"Quiet your body": a verbal cue to encourage a child to slow down or be still when a particular activity is not appropriate or safe.

"Safety first": above all things, we endeavor to keep children safe when they are at school. While this refers primarily to physical safety, it includes emotional and psychological safety as well.

"Slow down like a caterpillar": this is a verbal cue to remind a child to slow down and be in control of their body. It employs an image that is very concrete and real to any child that has observed the movement of a caterpillar, and additionally engages their imagination and creativity.

"Time-out/calm-down chair": this refers to a specific chair situated in each classroom that is designed as a place for a child to go to calm themselves and gain control over their behavior. It is not a punishment, but rather a structured and familiar place in which children feel safe and can begin to more independently internalize a sense of stopping in their bodies. It thus allows them to have difficult feelings and gain a sense of being able to manage them without feeling out of control. It is also a place in which they can reflect on their behavior and, with a teacher's help, develop a language with which they can discuss ways to change behavior or feelings that are problematic.

"Changes and goodbyes": a way to talk about changes in the school or home environment. Giving labels to changes, including goodbyes, can help the child identify feelings and emotions that often correlate with these events and develop coping strategies.

"School and home work together": this is a reminder to the child that their two worlds of home and school are working together to make the world a more consistent, predictable and integrated place in which the child can feel held and do the work (emotional and academic) that they need to do.

"School and home are a team, and you are part of the team": use of a sports metaphor to convey unity between home and school.

"Be a good friend": when a child is having a difficult time, they may attempt to take it out on a peer. They may not have strong social awareness, and engage in behavior that is not very caring or respectful of their peers. This phrase is used to cue a child that what they are doing or saying may be hurtful or disrespectful to another. It assumes that children have the capacity to relate in a friendly manner and encourages them to be aware of and work on doing so consistently. The other children of the group also feel protected and held in the relationship with their teachers and peers.

"Listen to your friends": this can serve to help a child listen to feedback or advice from their peers. It helps children perceive that others may have had similar experiences and have learned from them.

"Staying separate": often a child can get lost in the feelings or behavior of those around them (their friends, family members, etc.). This phrase serves as a reminder to maintain a boundary between what is really their own experience and that of another. For example, if a peer is having a difficult time and is becoming enraged, this cue helps a child to "stay separate" from the other child's anger and not become angry themselves or take it personally (when they are not involved). This is often difficult for children who are overwhelmed by their own or another's affect.

"Stay with me/be with me/be with people/be in the moment": these phrases can be used to help children "get out of their heads" and pay attention, but more explicitly connects that process to the relationship they have with a teacher/therapist. When a child is lost in his/her thoughts or fantasy, tuning in to the real world and what is happening in the moment can ground them in a physical and social reality that helps contain or hold their thoughts.

"Not being real/pretending/being in the real world": these are phrases that help a child distinguish between thoughts and behaviors that are real or shared and between real-world experiences versus ones that are related to fantasy or remain "in their head." Often children cannot make this distinction and need guidance and teaching to discriminate between the two so that they have a better grasp of another person's experience.

"Quiet your thoughts": this serves as a cue to help a child slow down and contain their thinking. It relates directly to the experience of stopping their bodies and staying safe, indicating that they can also begin to have control over what they think and thus develop strategies to "hold" their thoughts in a safe manner.

"Something you're working on": used to acknowledge a previously discussed area in which a child is struggling. As such, it reminds the child of the previous discussion, identifies a particular behavior as related to that discussion, and acknowledges that it is a process that takes time. It also helps a child take a perspective on the behavior (avoid getting caught up in the struggle but be able to step back and think about it with someone's help).

"Stuck": identifies when a child is having difficulty letting go of a thought or behavior that is inappropriate or getting in the way of them functioning socially, emotionally, or academically. It is a reminder to move on and connects the thought or behavior to previous discussions.

"A mixed bag of feelings": feelings that are all mixed up and difficult to sort out. It can also refer to a state in which more than one feeling is appropriately being felt and still needs to be acknowledged as complex and made up of different identifiable feelings.

"Being the boss of your feelings": this cues children to be in control of their feelings. It encourages the idea that feelings do not need to overwhelm an individual, but rather serve a purpose. It is intended to help children experience their feelings in a safe way without being overwhelmed by strong emotion. The goal is to teach them to make a relationship with their feelings in which they perceive themselves as being in charge and not helpless.

"'Giving' your mad feelings to someone": often, when children are overwhelmed or frightened by their own strong feelings they will attempt to get someone else to express what they are feeling for them. Instead of directly saying they are angry, for example, they will engage in behavior that will trigger anger in someone else. In this way, they feel in control of the feeling without having the experience of it or without having to acknowledge to themselves or others how they are really feeling.

"Good feeling": a feeling that is pleasant or desirable to experience (e.g., happy, pleased, proud, funny, strong, or smart).

"Having a hard time": a general term used to acknowledge the difficulty a child is having at any particular moment when it is not clear what the child is feeling or what the source of the difficulty is.

"Hurt feelings": how one feels when someone else has said or done something mean or without caring.

"Taking out your feelings on . . . ": when overwhelmed by one or more feelings, a child will often direct the feeling at someone inappropriately (i.e., someone unrelated to the cause of the feeling). This cue redirects the child who is experiencing the feeling and helps them think about why they are feeling a certain way and with whom they need to address this feeling.

"Too-big/too-silly feelings . . . ": acting in a way that suggests a child is escalating and is having difficulty modulating feelings. It may connote some level of anxiety that is being expressed with "silly" behavior.

"Use your words": often children will try to communicate their distress or struggle through behavior that is not appropriate or that is unclear. This cue serves to remind them that language can be a much more effective means of communication and that, more importantly, the relationship they have with a teacher, therapist, or parent can serve as the vehicle for the child to make the connection between their behavior or feelings and the words they need to express them.

"You can have your feelings in a safe way": a verbal cue that reassures children that even when they are having feelings that feel overwhelming or unsafe, the teachers will help them to stay safe while they are having them.

"You need to stop": a verbal reminder to immediately stop the unsafe or inappropriate behavior in which the child is engaged.

–7–

Facilitating Academic Instruction

Introduction

Within the school environment, academic achievement is largely measured by an individual's ability to develop skills within three major domains: reading, mathematics, and written expression. Neuropsychological testing of academic achievement, therefore, focuses on these three areas. Results from testing can be used to better understand an individual's relative academic strengths and vulnerabilities and as a means to develop more effective interventions and facilitate growth.

In this chapter, we focus on the development of academic skills from preschool through high school. Difficulties in any of the three spheres can be observed in the classroom when considered within the context of normal development. To that end, the tables below track the development of reading, math, and writing skills beginning in preschool through adolescence. They also include the evaluation tools most frequently used by neuropsychologists. For a more in-depth consideration of assessment tools, see Reinstein and Burau (2014).

While there may be many observational markers within the classroom suggesting that a child may be having difficulty in any one or some combination of these academic areas, focused testing is the most reliable means to identify the source of the difficulties and guide intervention. It must also be remembered that while difficulties in any of these arenas may be due to specific underlying neurologically based vulnerabilities, a lack of progress could also be due to other factors. For example, emergent literacy skills in preschoolers were correlated with behavior problems and attention deficits (Lonigan et al., 1999) as well as secure attachment (Bus & van Ijzendoorn, 1988). Therefore, an understanding of the whole child is essential in determining the underlying cause of a child's lack of academic progress (Reinstein & Burau, 2014). With that in mind, the following section provides a look at the behaviors that might be observed which would suggest a child is struggling with an underlying academic issue.

Observing Academic Functioning

Often a child's struggle with neurologically based academic vulnerabilities is not obvious and may manifest behaviorally and emotionally. It is rare, for example, that a child is aware of her own difficulties and even rarer that she could articulate why she is struggling. Consequently, one has to carefully observe and interpret certain behaviors as a communication about that struggle. It is not particularly helpful to merely describe a child's behavior as a means to gain attention or avoid a task. Rather, seeking attention or avoiding a task should be considered a child's attempt to tell a teacher or parent that she is finding the task too difficult. It is then the responsibility of the adult to interpret that behavior and begin to ask questions about what may underlie avoidance of or resistance to a particular task. In that light, the following observations of a child's behavior are likely indications that further questioning and evaluating are indicated.

- For example, one might suspect a child is having difficulty with written expression if the child readily engages in reading activities but resists writing tasks by engaging in behaviors such as:
  - slowly sharpening multiple pencils,
  - going to the bathroom and spending a long time there,
  - making frequent trips to get a drink of water,
  - pretending to think about what to write for an inordinate amount of time,
  - organizing materials for an extended period,
  - starting an unrelated conversation with a teacher or peer,
  - complaining of a somatic symptom (nausea, headache, eyes hurting, hand hurting),
  - suddenly becoming angry/sad/confused/silly for no apparent reason,
  - picking a fight with a peer, and
  - multiple erasures or ripping of paper.

These are only some within the possible range of behaviors that a teacher (or a parent regarding homework) might observe. These behaviors could manifest just as easily for children who are struggling with reading or math. Specifically, in respect to difficulties with written output, the questions one might then ask relate to a variety of possible causes for one or more of these behaviors. For example:

- Is the child avoiding writing because the mechanics/graphomotor skills are too difficult? Is this dysgraphia?
- Is the child having difficulty with the organization of written production such as sequencing of ideas, etc.? Is this an executive functioning problem?
- Is the child struggling to maintain a rate of output that matches a significant facility in language processing? Is this due to a significant discrepancy between strong language skills and a much slower processing speed?

- Is the child struggling to retrieve words? Is this a memory problem?
- Is the child having difficulty keeping ideas, instructions in her head? Is this a working memory problem?
- Is the child too easily distracted by happenings around her? Is this an attentional problem?
- Is the child distracted by internal thoughts or feelings? Is this an emotional problem related to events in the classroom or at home? Has the topic she is tasked to write about brought up distracting thoughts?
- Is the child having difficulty writing because they can't sit still or maintain an appropriate posture to engage in writing for any length of time? Is this a sensory/motor issue?

These are only some of the questions one might formulate as an initial attempt to understand a child's behavior as communication around a written expression problem. Some of the questions one might ask regarding reading difficulties might look like the following:

- Does a young child have difficulty rhyming words?
- Does the child consistently have difficulty sounding out words or confuse letters and sounds?
- Does the child have difficulty breaking down words into parts?
- Does the child prefer books with a preponderance of pictures over text?
- Does the child gravitate towards books that are much lower than her grade level?
- Does the child decode words adequately but can't explain what she's read?
- Is reading aloud slow and effortful?
- Is spelling poor?

The following are some questions one might ask related to concerns about mathematics skills development:

- Does the child have difficulty or is she slow in recalling basic math facts, rules, formulas, or steps?
- Is the child's math production imprecise?
- Does the child have difficulty discerning/remembering patterns?
- Is the child having difficulty sequencing steps?
- Is the child overwhelmed by many problems on one sheet?
- Does the child have difficulty deciding what is/is not important in word problems?
- Does the child have difficulty switching between operations in complex problems?
- Does the child have difficulty translating word problems into math operations?
- Does the child have difficulty organizing more complex operations spatially on the page?
- Does the child have difficulty understanding what a three-dimensional object might look like from a different perspective?

The above are just some of the observations and questions one might ask as a means to better understand why a child might be engaging in some of the behaviors described previously. Depending on the specific set of observations one might make, a more focused evaluation could be indicated. Most importantly, however, these behaviors must be understood within the context of a child's attempt to communicate important information to those around her. Interpreting these behaviors as laziness, attitude, or just opposition is never helpful.

Academic Skill Development

The following tables chart the typical development of reading, written expression, and mathematics skills over a child's lifespan from preschool to high school. The assessment tools employed to evaluate academic achievement in each of these areas and at each developmental stage are included as well. It is important to note that these developmental trajectories relate to English speakers within a western culture. The development of these skills may differ for children speaking other languages or for those who have been raised in other countries.

TABLE 7.1 Reading Skill Development

Age	*Skills*	*Assessment Tools*
Emerging pre-reader (4–6 years old)	• Child "pretends" to read • Child retells a story looking at pages in book previously read to him/her • Child names letters of alphabet • Child recognizes some signs • Child can print own name • Child plays with books, pencils, paper • Child understands thousands of words but can read few, if any	• RAN/RAS – assesses child's ability to recognize a visual symbol such as a letter/color and name it accurately and rapidly • Comprehensive Test of Phonological Processing (CTOPP-2) – assesses child's phonological awareness, phonological memory, and rapid naming skills • Wechsler Individual Achievement Test, Third Edition (WIAT-III) – subtests evaluate phonological, decoding, fluency, and comprehension skills • WJ-IV Ach – subtests evaluate phonological, decoding, fluency, and comprehension skills • Kaufman Test of Educational Achievement 3 (K-TEA-3) – subtests evaluate phonological, decoding, fluency, and comprehension skills

(continued)

TABLE 7.1 *(continued)*

Age	*Skills*	*Assessment Tools*
Novice reader (6–7 years old)	• Child is learning relationship between letters and sounds and between printed and spoken words • Child starts to read simple text containing high-frequency words and phonically regular words • Child sounds out new one-syllable words • Child receives direct instruction in letter–sound relations • Child is being read to on level above what he/she can read independently • Child can understand up to 4,000 words when heard and can read about 600	• RAN/RAS • CTOPP-2 • WIAT-III • WJ-IV Ach • K-TEA-3 • Gray Oral Reading Test 5 (GORT-5) – assesses oral reading fluency and comprehension • Gray Silent Reading Test (GSRT) – assesses silent reading fluency and comprehension
Decoding reader (7–9 years old)	• Child is reading simple and familiar stories with increasing fluency • Child is consolidating basic decoding elements, sight vocabulary, and meaning in familiar stories • Child is receiving direct instruction in advanced decoding • Child is receiving direct instruction in reading of family and interesting materials • Child is being read to at levels above independent reading level to develop language, vocabulary, and concepts • Child knows about 9,000 words when heard and can read 3,000	• RAN/RAS • CTOPP-2 • WIAT-III • WJ-IV Ach • K-TEA-3 • GORT-5 • GSRT
Fluent, comprehending reader (9–15 years old)	• Reading is used to learn new ideas, gain knowledge, experience new feelings, learn new attitudes, and explore issues from different perspectives • Reading includes study of textbooks, reference works, trade books, magazines, and newspapers containing unfamiliar vocabulary and syntax • There is a systematic study of word meaning • Child is guided through text by discussions, answering questions, generating questions, writing, etc. • Listening comprehension is still more efficient than reading comprehension until the end of this stage when, for some, reading may be more efficient	• RAN/RAS • CTOPP-2 • WIAT-III • WJ-IV Ach • K-TEA-3 • GORT-5 • GSRT

Expert reader (16 years and older)	• Readers are making inferences while reading by generating hypotheses and integrating information into knowledge base • Individual is reading widely from broad range of complex materials (sciences, humanities, politics, current affairs) • Reading comprehension is better than listening comprehension of difficult materials	• RAN/RAS • CTOPP-2 • WIAT-III • WJ-IV Ach • K-TEA-3 • GORT-5 • GSRT

Source: Wolf (2008).

TABLE 7.2 Writing Skill Development

Stage	*Skills*	*Assessment Tools*
Literacy roots (4–6 years) **Stage 1**	• Awareness of functions and purposes of reading and writing • Developing knowledge of the world • Developing phonological awareness • Developing grapheme awareness • Understands concepts of books	• WIAT-III – subtests assess spelling, fluency, and grammar • WJ-IV Ach – subtests assess fluency, spelling, and grammar • K-TEA-3 – subtests assess spelling and grammar
Initial literacy (6–7 years) **Stage 2**	• Child makes non-alphabetic markings believing it is writing • Spellers partially recognize that letters stand for sounds • Writers can represent all sounds phonetically (some letter choices do not conform to conventional spelling) • Writers recognize that words have particular morphological structures, not just phonological features • Spellers show greater knowledge of orthographic system	• WIAT-III – subtests assess spelling, fluency, and grammar • WJ-IV Ach – subtests assess fluency, spelling, and grammar • K-TEA-3 – subtests assess spelling and grammar
Confirmation, fluency, ungluing (7–8 years) **Stage 3**	• Consolidation of earlier learning • Knowledge access becomes more fluent or automatic • Many words read at sight and written at will • Greater effort to use bigger words • Higher level of knowledge about graphophonics, the morphological patterns in complex words	• WIAT-III – subtests assess spelling, grammar, theme development, and text organization of an essay • WH-IV Ach – subtests assess fluency, spelling, grammar, and thematic content of an essay • K-TEA-3 – subtests assess spelling, grammar, and thematic content of an essay

(continued)

TABLE 7.2 *(continued)*

Stage	*Skills*	*Assessment Tools*
Writing for learning the new (9–13 years) **Stage 4**	• Meaning becomes focus of writing • Increase in abstract content, new ideas, and new vocabulary • Increase in more complex syntactical structure • Increased ability to create and use word meanings and meaningful connected text for multiple purposes	• Test of Written Language (TOWL-4) – subtests assess orthographic and grammatical conventions as well as thematic content • WIAT-III • WJ-IV Ach • K-TEA-3
Multiple viewpoints (14–18 years) **Stage 5**	• Elaboration of Stage 4 skills • Increased awareness of one's own comprehension and meaning production • Enriched understanding of text structure and its use for effect • Ability to take different perspectives • Emergence of critical thinking skills allows for self-monitoring and revision to accommodate audience	• TOWL-4 • WIAT-III • WJ-IV Ach • K-TEA-3
Construction and reconstruction (18 and older) **Stage 6**	• Movement from an understanding of knowledge as factual to the conception of knowledge as subjective • Increased understanding of how readers and writers interact	• TOWL-4 • WIAT-III • WJ-IV Ach • K-TEA-3

Source: Fitzgerald & Shanahan (2000).

TABLE 7.3 Mathematical Skill Development

Age	*Skills*	*Assessment Tools*
Preschool **3–5 years**	• Beginning at 2 years, children are developing an understanding of number concepts and counting • 3- to 4-year-olds know number words in sequence from 1–10 • 3- to 4-year-olds begin to associate number words with specific small quantities • Understanding of ordinal relationships for small quantities (equivalent, greater than, less than) • Sense that addition increases and subtraction decreases quantity (arithmetic) for quantities less than 4	• WIAT-III – subtests assess math concepts, calculation, and fluency skills • WJ-IV Ach – subtests assess math concepts, calculation, and fluency skills • K-TEA-3 – subtests assess math concepts and calculation

5–7 years	• Understanding of number concepts and counting continues to improve • 5-year-olds begin to understand concept of cardinality (last number counted is equivalent to the total number) • 5-year-olds understand order of counting items (left to right, right to left) doesn't alter end result • Gradual development of ordinal relationships for larger numbers • Understanding of arithmetic gradually increases • Kindergarten children are able to solve simple change (action performed by child) and combine (static relationship) word problems • By 7 years, most children know number words up to 100	• WIAT-III • WJ-IV Ach • K-TEA-3
7–8 years	• Understanding of number concepts and counting continues to improve • Understand that each number can be represented by groups of other numbers • Able to use numbers for measurement • Concept of cardinality is more consistent • Development of ordinal relationships for larger numbers continues • 8-year-olds develop mature number knowledge and counting skills • Second-grade children are able to solve most compare/contrast word problems (e.g., greater than/less than)	• WIAT-III • WJ-IV Ach • K-TEA-3
9–10 years	• 9-year-olds apply quantitative procedures (e.g., ruler) to make simple measurements • Third-grade children solve simpler equalize word problems (action taken to make two sets equal)	• WIAT-III • WJ-IV Ach • K-TEA-3
11–18 years	• Sixth-grade children solve difficult equalize word problems • Development of algebra skills begins in middle school through high school and depends on ability to translate language into algebraic variables and development of metacognitive skills • Continued development depends on problem-solving strategies, underlying memory representations, and abstract schema-based knowledge • Mathematical skills continue to develop with a distinction between numerical facility (arithmetic) and mathematical reasoning (mathematical problem-solving) and are influenced by genetics • Education continues to be the strongest influence on math skills development	• WIAT-III • WJ-IV Ach • K-TEA-3

Source: Geary (1994).

Creating a Group Holding Environment

In Chapter 6 we discussed how the teacher and the relationships he or she develops with students are major factors in the creation of the classroom holding environment. To varying degrees, each student relies on an educational environment in which learning can take place safely and securely. Whether or not a student likes or dislikes a teacher, the student must trust that, as a student, they will be free from harm. An environment in which a student feels disliked or, worse, physically, psychologically, or emotionally threatened by a teacher or classmate, does not facilitate academic progress. Furthermore, different students may rely to different degrees on the nature of the relationship they establish with the teachers, with some needing more emotional nurturing than others. It is the role of the teacher to perceive the needs of the students they teach and to establish the most appropriate relationship that is *good enough* to provide the type of holding environment that a particular student needs. On a larger scale, however, the holding environment must extend beyond each individual relationship to encompass the kind of holding the whole classroom needs. To do so on the teacher's part requires awareness and consideration of what goes into holding the group so that the group's academic progress can be ensured. As Riley (2011) has noted:

> The traditionally conceived foundations of education, the 3Rs (Reading, writing, and arithmetic), are not the foundations at all. In fact they can only be built on an even more fundamental set of 3Rs; relationships (Relationship from the student's perspective, Relationship from the teacher's perspective, and the priority given to Relationship formation and maintenance from school leadership). For a school to function effectively and for students to learn effectively both sets of 3Rs must be in place.
>
> (p. 1)

So then, how does one establish a good enough holding environment for the classroom that is fundamentally based on relationships but also includes the teacher's use of the actual physical, temporal, and social environment that serves as an extension of those relationships? This was a question posed by the developmental psychologist Urie Bronfenbrenner as he considered the relationship between the physical environment and relationships over the time course of an individual's development (e.g., Bronfenbrenner & Evans, 2000).

As all teachers would agree, a certain amount of structure within the classroom environment is necessary to facilitate academic growth. For most children, this includes an organized physical space, a schedule that organizes time, and a level of consistency in the relationships between teachers and students, as well as with peers, established within that context.

The physical environment of the classroom should be one in which children feel both held comfortably and stimulated. Research suggests that it is best to begin the year with greater structure, clear expectations, and a focus on socialization, and then work towards more independence (Emmer et al., 1980). Groupings in respect to age, ability, capacity for collaboration, and peer tutoring is also important to consider (Wilczenski et al., 2001).

To facilitate these processes, it is important to consider the spatial organization of seating for whole-group instruction and the creation of areas to increase small-group instruction or a quiet space. It is also helpful to designate a library and select materials to post on bulletin boards that are engaging but not distracting. Materials for student use in the classroom should be organized neatly, labeled, color-coded, and kept to a minimum. Clear expectations of how materials should be used should be displayed prominently. Establishing routines for entering the classroom, ending activities, transitioning between activities, refocusing students' attention, responding to questions, handing in work, and ending the day all provide a level of consistency and predictability that facilitates instruction. Previewing curriculum and the scheduled time for various units by providing weekly agendas, recording parts of lessons on a board and crossing them off when finished, or scheduling activities for free time, give students a sense of being held. Refocusing techniques that are well established and part of the classroom's overall identity can also help reinforce a sense of group cohesion (Carty, 2000).

A consideration and focus on all of the above areas are just some of the ways that help to create an environment in which students feel held in space and time as well as within peer and teacher relationships. A teacher's sensitivity to the needs of the students as a group provides those students with a sense of being seen and cared for and facilitates the learning process through an appreciation of the relationships they establish.

To summarize, here are some tips on building a classroom space and group that facilitates a holding environment:

- Post a schedule and do your best to follow it. Discuss changes in the schedule in advance if you can.
- Develop classroom routines for managing materials, starting work time, and transitions. Do group activities that promote social cohesion.
- Provide each child with a space for their materials that is theirs. Also provide a space that is for the group (bulletin board).
- Consider how to use the space. Make sure you have an area for larger group instruction, areas for small-group instruction, and individual private spaces as well.
- Keep the physical space organized and clutter-free.
  Preview lessons, provide weekly agendas, and help students track where they are in their academic projects.

Chapter 7 Appendix: Facilitating Academic Instruction

USING ART TO ESTABLISH GROUP RAPPORT

Goal: Foster connection between students while recognizing individual differences.

Materials: Large (several feet x several feet depending on how much bulletin board space is available) piece of semi-thick paper, acrylic paint in a variety of colors, large paint brushes, large space that can get messy (art room or outdoor space), scissors and construction paper for making a frame, images of paintings by Jackson Pollock, painting smocks or space shirts/pants.

Directions: Show images of paintings by Jackson Pollock to the classroom. Discuss how he was the first person to ever create art in this way. Suggest to the class that, as a group, we will make our own Pollock painting. Each student is allowed to choose (or make) a color of their very own to represent who they are. Take the class to the art room or an outdoor space and demonstrate how to drizzle, splatter, and drop paint onto the large piece of paper. One at a time, the students are invited to drizzle their color onto the group painting. Make sure one color does not dominate but that each student can be represented by their color. Have students help clean the paint brushes and space if needed. Once the painting has dried, cut out one large piece of the painting to frame and hang in the classroom. Cut smaller versions of the painting for students to take home with them.

COLLABORATIVE RULE DEVELOPMENT

Goal: Engage students in developing their own community, expectations, and means for holding each other accountable. Some rules are determined by the teacher in order to set a specific tone as teacher and group leader.

Materials: Large pieces of paper, markers.

Directions: At the beginning of the academic year, have a discussion with students to develop a set of rules. Provide examples if necessary. Start with rule 1: safety first. Explain to the students that this means physical, emotional, and psychological safety is a top priority. Ask them how to make sure they each feel safe. After that, ask the students for more suggestions on how they want to be treated by each other. To start, keep the list of rules relatively short to avoid overwhelming the students. Make it clear that this is a working document and rules can be added to it. Also establish that while their ideas are valuable, as the teacher you will decide if a rule is appropriate.

Attempt to word rules positively. For example, "Don't interrupt without permission" could be phrased as, "Raise your hand to get attention from the teacher and friends." This gives the student clear expectations and coping skills.

If appropriate, also discuss consequences of breaking the rules and apply consequences fairly and consistently. If the classroom is using time-out, this could be a good time to discuss the meaning and purpose of time-out.

Be sure to display the rules and consequences in an appropriate space. Encourage the students to either sign or decorate the rules. This ensures that they all know and understand the rules and agree to abide by them.

Make sure the conversation is age-appropriate. This can be done as young as kindergarten, but keep the discussion shorter to match their attention span.

Adaptations: If students are reluctant to share their ideas, they can write or draw them on a piece of paper and turn it in to the teacher.

Based on: Canter, L. (2001).

FACILITATING TRANSITIONS AND DEVELOPING ROUTINE

There are many classroom activities that can benefit from the development of routine and clear expectations. Routines for these activities may take time for the students to learn, but the creation of expectations ensures the students don't need to problem-solve in the moment in order to complete simple tasks. This lightens the load on their working memory and processing speed. Building routines relies on their long-term and implicit memory. Once the routine is established, it saves time. Here is a list of classroom activities that can benefit from establishing a routine. Note, they vary depending on setting (public school) or grade level (formatting papers may not be required of first-graders). Also, start to think of each of these things as a transition. Every one of them involves either moving from one space to another, engaging in new materials, or shifting focus from one thing to something else. Imagine each of these transitions as a tiny gap that can be filled with emotional or behavioral distress.

Entering the classroom	Saying "Please" and "Thank you"
Getting to work immediately	Suddenly becoming ill
Arriving late/being tardy	Receiving visitors to the room
Ending the class period/dismissal	Responding to a severe weather alert
Listening to/responding to questions	Responding to a fire drill
Participating in class discussions	Asking a question
Needing a pencil or paper	Returning to a task after an interruption
Keeping your desk orderly	Finishing a test or assignment early
Checking out classroom materials	Moving about the room
Indicating whether you understand	Handing out materials
Coming to attention	Getting materials without disturbing others
Returning after an absence	Passing in papers
Working cooperatively	Finding directions for each assignment
Changing groups	Returning student work
Keeping your notebook	Keeping a progress report
Going to the office	Knowing the schedule for the day/class
Requesting help or information	Formatting papers/appropriate heading
Going to the library/career center	Listening to an announcement over the intercom or TV
Using passes to be out of the classroom during class time	
Behaving when the teacher is out of the classroom or when a substitute teacher is present	

The first step in facilitating transitions is to think carefully about the number of transitions you require in a given time period. Are they all necessary? Can some of them be cut out? Does the schedule allow time for transition? How might individual children or students need specific support during each transition? It is important to start developing routines for transitions and classroom activities on the first day of school. This way the students (and the teacher) do not need to unlearn bad habits. Learning how to be in the classroom and how to be together is the first objective.

Prior to starting any transition, prepare the students with a warning that is verbal, auditory (like a bell or chime), and maybe even visual. This could look like a sand glass, or a sand glass counting down. Remind the group what is coming next in the schedule. If students don't have time to complete what they are currently working on, let them know when their next opportunity will be. Provide positive feedback once they stop the activity.

Recognize that different groups of students will need help with transitions in different ways. For example, some groups of third-graders can line up when asked to line up. They will stand calmly and wait for the next direction. Others need to be called one by one to get into line. The order they are called on could be based on their behavior or whether they look ready to calmly line up, according to how they will walk past each other in order to get to line, or who they can successfully stand beside. Let the students know that it is a goal for them to independently line up. Give them a set of expectations so they know how to behave. While this sounds serious, it can also be done playfully, saying their names in a silly way or having some sort of song that goes along with the activity. Some groups might do best if told to strike a pose like a statue while standing in line. Transitions can be structured and fun! Once everyone is lined up, praise the group for meeting your expectation.

Imagine a classroom taking a break to get water and a snack. All at once, the students rush out of their chairs and head for their backpacks. Some groups can independently manage this transition. Other groups need more structure or else the room bursts into chaos. Start each academic year providing structure and work towards less structure. For example, at the beginning of the year, allow four students at a time to go to their backpack; meanwhile, the other students can look at a book or other material related to the last lesson. Once the four students have returned to their seats, instruct the next four to put away their books and get their snack, etc.

An important aspect of teaching a group how to transition is to recognize how many steps are required for each transition. Make a verbal and visual chart to support the children who cannot remember multi-step directions. *Do* the transition with them to model appropriate behavior. If you are tending to another matter, such as organizing lesson materials, the group may not feel held in a relationship and may quickly stray from direction. Once a routine is well established, it may be possible that the routine will hold them and so the teacher can attend to other matters. In some cases, the students can take turns facilitating transitions once they have been learned.

It is also important to recognize when you are meeting the needs of the group versus when you are meeting your own needs. There is a time and place for both, but the group usually comes first.

Imagine a classroom coming in from lunch or recess. They are chattering, distracted by the previous activity, and not yet engaged in classroom behavior. The challenge here is to harness the energy so they coalesce as a group with a common goal. In these moments, it could be useful to create a group challenge. Perhaps time them as a group to see how quickly they can settle into their seats. Set a standard for what it looks like to be ready: (1) sit in your seat quietly, (2) get out a pencil or pen, and (3) do not talk with your neighbor. Once they invest in the "race," they can encourage each other. At random, reward smooth transitions with a fun activity and planned break or a brief outing. While energy is high, perhaps engage them in a group movement activity related to the lesson that is being taught to help facilitate their regulation.

Groups benefit from learning what a transition is. Help the students identify various transitions throughout the day and week. If there are specific transitions that tend to be more difficult, point them out, set expectations and goals (if the students can participate in this, all the better), and provide extra structure. Developing awareness of how each individual contributes to the group transition can be empowering. Make sure not to shame slower people. Create peers that can help each other. Foster strengths and always provide accurate feedback. If the group did not successfully complete a transition or meet your expectations, do not say that they did. Instead, mention that they need to continue to work on transitions and give specific feedback/ instructions on how to improve. Once they do, then give praise.

Based on: Ostrosky et al. (n.d.).

DEVELOPING A GROUP BEHAVIOR PLAN FOR CLASSROOM MANAGEMENT

There are many types of group behavioral plans. They can focus on how an individual performs within a group. There could be a group token economy in which all students work to earn something independently and get a reward. There could be a plan that makes one student the class "hero," even if temporarily. The type of plan focused on here is intended to develop group cohesion by having peers support one another and share a common goal.

First, determine what skill the group needs to develop (such as making a smooth transition, having quiet study time, or supporting each other). Secondly, find a group reward that most students would enjoy. It is best if this is an activity that will foster further connection, not individual toys or prizes. Various types of parties (dance party, movie party) could be utilized or extra time outside could be provided. Perhaps a special outing such as sledding (if you're in a cold climate) or a trip to the local library might be appropriate. Third, carefully define the group behavior to clarify your expectations. For example, perhaps the group has a tendency to be very negative about various activities throughout the day. Find a way to define the negative comments. For example, refer to them as "negativity bombs." Help the students see how the negative comments impact each other and make it harder to complete goals or accomplish a task. Each time a student engages in a negativity bomb, make an explosion noise with your mouth and mime an explosion going off. Now that the behavior is defined for yourself and the group, count the number of negativity bombs that occur in one day and write down the number. This is the baseline. Challenge the group to reduce the baseline. Set a number that feels appropriate and achievable. Once they achieve the number, have the party as promised. Provide praise in each period in which there are no negativity bombs. Encourage the students to support each other. If someone sets off a negativity bomb and others shame them, it is a double bomb. If someone makes a positive comment, encourage them to praise each other. Make a chart or visual to help the students and you track their progress. This should be prominently displayed in the classroom and easy for you to access so you can add to it in the moment, thus providing immediate feedback.

You could also counter the negativity by developing a similar plan that encourages the students to support and help each other. In this way, you are ameliorating the undesired group behavior and encouraging a desirable behavior.

This is an example of how to define a problem within a group and address it. The group reward must be worth their effort or they will not want to reach the goal.

Based on: Maag (2001).

TEACHING STUDENT BEHAVIOR

Goal: Help students learn behaviors and set expectations that are conducive to a learning environment.

Materials: Pencils, markers or crayons, Student Behavior Checklist (see next page), chime or bell (clapping works if you don't have a chime or bell).

Directions: Start a lesson by telling students there are certain ways of behaving that help most people learn. Tell them this is a time to practice those behaviors. One by one, review the items on the Student Behavior Checklist. For example, number one, "Sit up in your chair." Have the students sit in their chair the way you expect them to and then play "opposite day." Instruct the students to flop on the table, sit on the floor, or sag in their seat when you ring the bell. Turn number one "Sit up in your chair" into a Simon Says-style game. Move on to the next item and repeat the same "game." Check the box for each behavior as you go down the list. This will help set expectations for future lessons and generate a baseline to operate from. In the future, if students are having a hard time engaging in the expected behavior, make jokes about "opposite day" or even play the game briefly to help them reach an appropriate arousal level.

Adaptations:

- If students have special chairs, seats, cushions, etc., that allow them to sit in their most optimal way (usually with the consultation of an OT), allow the chair and integrate it into the game. If they have other sensory difficulties or physical disabilities that don't allow them to participate in the list as it is made, develop a list that is individualized to them.
- Tape the list (or an abbreviated version of it) to the students' desks. Reference the list at the beginning of lessons to ensure they are ready. If at some point during the lesson they veer from the expected student behavior, cue them by tapping on the list.
- If a student continues to struggle, use an outline of a body and ask them to help explain why participating in the expected behavior is difficult. They can color it in, draw over it, or talk about it.
- If a student has difficulty reading, make a Student Behavior Checklist using visual symbols only.

Student Behavior Checklist

☐ 1. Sit up in your chair.

☐ 2. Look at the teacher.

☐ 3. Listen to the teacher.

☐ 4. Think about your work.

☐ 5. Do not talk while you are reading or writing.

☐ 6. Pay attention to your work.

☐ 7. No chatting during work time.

TAKING CARE OF THE CLASSROOM AS A GROUP

Goal: Facilitate community and purpose, highlighting that each student can contribute to the classroom environment. Also, transfer some responsibility to students for keeping the classroom running smoothly, resulting in uninterrupted instruction.

Materials: Make a chart (or use a pocket chart) that outlines all of the classroom jobs you will require the class to complete. Have a piece of paper or token that represents each student.

Directions: Prior to the school year, make a list of all the jobs you would like the students to complete. Make the job title sound fun or mature. Choose an appropriate number of jobs and save some to add or swap in later in the year when other routines have been established. Decide if you want the students to do jobs alone or in pairs. Also decide how frequently you want the jobs to rotate: once a day, once a week, once a month, etc.

On the first day of school, introduce the job chart. Tell the students that during the first week of school, we will all practice each job together and that in the next week they will each be assigned a job. Explain how the chart works and prominently display it in the classroom near the schedule.

Be sure that your schedule allows time to review the jobs and their daily completion. Often, review can happen during a morning check-in when the daily schedule is being covered. Anticipate that at the beginning of the year, jobs will take longer to complete. In older classrooms that are subjects (Science, for example), jobs can still be effective, even for one period. At the beginning of class, review who is responsible for cleaning or organizing different materials.

In order for classroom jobs to be successful, they must be integrated into the routine and used/enforced consistently. It can also be helpful to occasionally, without notice, reward the classroom for doing well with a classroom routine.

Adaptation: Allow the students to decorate the piece of paper with their name on it or make their token for the chart.

Based on: Wong et al. (2014).

Potential Jobs

Attendance Taker

Breakfast/Snack Helper

Bulletin Board Helper

Calendar Helper

Desk Inspector

Errand Runner

Floor Monitor (makes sure floor is clean)

Lights Monitor

Line Ender

Line Leader

Media Assistant (turns TV/computer off/on, volume)

Meteorologist (announces forecast)

Paper Passers/Collectors

Plant Waterer (Botanist)

Schedule Helper

Supply Passers

–8–

Development of the IEP

Introduction

In this chapter, we return to the story of Leila from Chapter 1 to demonstrate how the results of a comprehensive neuropsychological assessment can be used to develop an IEP. Then, various ways the results can be integrated into different sections of the IEP will be presented. This chapter assumes the reader has a basic understanding of the process of writing an IEP.

Case Study

Leila was a 9-year-old girl in third grade at a private school in the Boston Metro area. Her parents were well educated and she had a brother in first grade at the same school. Her development was remarkable for difficulty sleeping, fine motor delays, and sensory processing issues. Family history was significant for a reading disability, depression, and schizophrenia.

Leila began attending the same school just before she turned three. Over the course of her six years there, she had increased difficulty with modulation, aggression, following directions, transitions, rigidity, rudeness, and social awareness. Nevertheless, she was performing well academically. Previous testing documented very superior verbal and visual perceptual skills, high-average working memory abilities, and a superior processing speed on the WISC-IV. Leila's parents sought a new evaluation as a means not only to update her profile but, more importantly, address their concerns about her behavior.

Leila was evaluated over two three-and-a-half-hour sessions. Her speech was rapid, fluid, and articulate. She enthusiastically described a number of her interests in considerable detail but was able to transition to testing without difficulty. She evidenced a considerable amount of motor overflow, fidgeting, kicking the table rhythmically, placing her head on her arms, stretching, making propulsive sounds with her lips, and placing her fingers in her mouth or gently biting her hand or arm. She worked very quickly on virtually all of the tasks presented and, at times, she became impulsive in her attempt to answer quickly. She used a number of effective strategies, was very cooperative, worked hard, and attempted to do her best.

Leila's Verbal Comprehension skills fell in the Very Superior range (VCI = 133; 99th percentile) as did her Visual Spatial abilities (VSI = 135; 99th percentile) and Fluid Reasoning skills (FRI = 131; 98th percentile). While her Processing Speed Index fell in the Superior range (PSI = 123; 94th percentile), her Working Memory was at the lower end of the Average range (WMI = 97; 42nd percentile).

Leila's Verbal Comprehension Index (VCI) – a measure of her ability to access and apply acquired word knowledge, her Visual Spatial Index (VSI) – her ability to evaluate visual details and understand visual spatial relationships, her Fluid Reasoning Index (FRI) – an indication of her ability to identify and apply visual conceptual relationships, and her Processing Speed Index (PSI) – her ability to visually scan and organize a graphomotor output, were no different from each other. However, her Working Memory Index (WMI) – her ability to hold visual and auditory information on line while performing mental operations upon it – was significantly lower than the four other indices and thus represented a significant relative vulnerability. There was no significant difference between subtest scores in three of the areas (VCI, VSI, WMI), suggesting that her abilities within each of these domains were commensurate while there was a significant difference between subtest scores in two areas (FRI, PSI), suggesting that her skills in these areas were uneven.

On the Rey–Osterrieth Complex Figure Test, Leila scored at the 50th percentile on the Copy portion, below the 50th percentile on the Immediate Recall portion, and below the 25th percentile on the Delayed Recall portion. The demand for graphomotor precision and organization as well as the consolidation and recall of visual detail compromised her performance on this task. Furthermore, on a task of visual motor integration (the Beery VMI), she scored at the 9th percentile. In respect to executive functions, Leila's average working memory abilities were impacted by her variable attention and she had significant difficulty sustaining attention for low-interest tasks. She also struggled with impulsivity, distractibility, self-monitoring, self-correcting, cognitive flexibility, and planning. Her visual memory skills were superior, while her verbal memory skills were very superior. However, there was a decrement in her ability to recall visual detail over time. Leila's academic skills, academic fluency, and ability to apply academic skills were all in the average range, as were her broad math abilities. However, while her broad reading skills were high average, her broad written language skills were low average.

The graph (Figure 8.1) represents a standard bell curve with the scores from the tests of cognitive and academic functioning. It portrays the broad spread from the 9th percentile for Leila's visual motor skills to the 99.9th percentile for verbal recall.

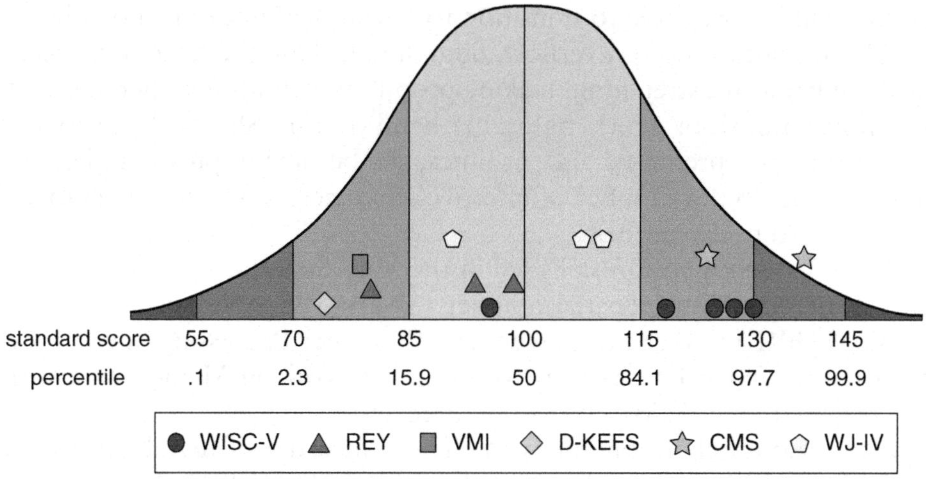

FIGURE 8.1 Assessment Results on the Bell Curve

On measures of behavioral functioning, Leila's parents reported Clinically Significant levels of concern regarding her Externalizing Problems and At-Risk levels of concern regarding Behavioral Symptoms. Leila's teacher reported Clinically Significant levels of concern regarding her Externalizing and Internalizing Problems as well as her Behavioral Symptoms. Furthermore, both parents and her teacher noted Clinically Significant levels of concern regarding Emotional Self-Control, Executive Functions, and Negative Emotionality as well as Hyperactivity and Aggression, while her teacher also noted Clinically Significant levels of concern regarding Depression, Atypicality, and Bullying. Leila reported a Clinically Significant level of concern about her Hyperactivity.

Tests of social perception indicated that Leila demonstrated an average ability to read and articulate most affective facial expressions, excepting anger, and an above-average ability to understand mental operations and take another's perspective within the context of a formal testing environment. However, her ability to carry out these operations in real time, when faced with challenging social situations, was often significantly compromised by her emotional state.

In respect to emotional functioning, Leila presented as an intellectually gifted young girl who was grounded in reality and who had the capacity to think logically and clearly. Difficulties with graphomotor precision and executive functions, particularly in respect to sustaining her attention, hyperactivity, impulsivity, distractibility, self-monitoring, switching cognitive set and planning, made it challenging for her to meet certain environmental demands. These factors had additionally contributed to Leila's difficulty tolerating frustration, emotional outbursts, and incidents of lashing out at others both physically and verbally. Because Leila had the capacity for self-awareness, she was acutely aware of the difficulty she was having both managing herself and within relationships. Consequently, she had gone on the defense and had attempted to cover up her vulnerabilities by appearing overconfident and inflating her self-worth. This tendency to distort had negatively impacted her relationships, a factor that had exacerbated her already existing limited social skills. These findings suggested that, without additional support to use her considerable strengths in a more productive manner, Leila was vulnerable to becoming more overwhelmed, feel negative about herself, be socially compromised, and feel anxious and depressed.

In summary, these results were consistent with the following diagnoses:

- Developmental Coordination Disorder,
- ADHD-Combined Presentation,
- Executive Dysfunction, and
- Mood Disorder NOS with features of anxiety and depression.

Means for Integrating Results

Results of the assessment can be integrated in a number of ways. First, the results must be included in the IEP document and discussed by the team. In this way, the results are used to *describe* the child's strengths and vulnerabilities. This is done in the first page of the document, in the Present Levels of Performance A (PLEP A) and PLEP B as well as in current performance levels on all the goals.

The results are also used to generate appropriate accommodations, interventions, and modifications for the student's school experience.

- *Accommodations* allow the student to fully access general educational curriculum without changing instructional content. Accommodations eliminate obstacles without changing or reducing the learning expectations.
- *Interventions* are skill-building strategies which are implemented and monitored to improve a targeted skill. This may involve changing instruction or adding to it.
- *Modifications* change, lower, or reduce (or increase in the case of gifted students) learning or assessment expectations. Results in learning are different from what other students of the same age and grade might produce.

Common Core State Standards

Before going any further in developing an IEP for Leila, it is important to briefly review the CCSS as they relate to the content of an IEP. In 2009, the National Governors Association and the Council of Chief State School Officers began to develop the CCSS, creating for the first time a set of standards that could be adopted by all states in order to provide a rigorous and consistent education across the country. In 2010, the CCSS was released, providing educators and parents with a map for instruction at each grade level that determined what knowledge and skills should be attained by the end of each grade. The CCSS have been adopted by 43 states, the District of Columbia, and four territories (Power-deFur, 2015). They are used for developing curriculum, providing benchmarks for academic assessment, and developing specific learning goals on IEPs.

The CCSS outline areas of curriculum that students, with or without learning disabilities, must have an opportunity to engage in so that they can develop skills necessary for success. To this end, IEPs can contain annual goals that align with and facilitate the attainment of grade-level academic standards (McNulty & Gloeckler, 2011). The student must also have services designed to meet their needs in order to access general curriculum (U.S. Department of Education, 2004). Students with significant cognitive disabilities may qualify for alternate assessments or require significant support to take standard RTI assessments that determine students' abilities to achieve grade-level performances based on the CSSS (McNulty & Gloeckler, 2011). The results of Leila's evaluation indicate that she is working at (or above) grade level in certain areas, but that her difficulties impact her ability to access the curriculum. As a result, the following IEP example focuses on the types of modifications and accommodations Leila might need in order to access the curriculum. If her struggles were related to specific learning difficulties and she was behind in grade level, goals might reference specific standards.

Present Levels of Performance A

PLEP A is used to describe the areas of educational curriculum that are impacted by an individual's difficulties. It addresses in what areas of education they will need accommodations, interventions, or modifications in order to access learning. A brief description of the child is presented. In the image below, it is indicated that Leila's difficulties, as documented in the evaluation results, impact all areas of learning. The brief paragraph specifies how Leila's difficulties impact her learning and provide a baseline for the frequency of learning disruption.

TABLE 8.1 IEP Example: PLEP A

<table>
<tr><td colspan="4">Present Levels of Educational Performance
A: General Curriculum</td></tr>
<tr><td colspan="2">Check all that apply.</td><td colspan="2"></td></tr>
<tr><td colspan="2"></td><td colspan="2">General curriculum area(s) affected by this student's disability(ies):</td></tr>
<tr><td>X</td><td>English Language Arts</td><td colspan="2">Consider the language, composition, literature (including reading) and media strands</td></tr>
<tr><td>X</td><td>History and Social Sciences</td><td colspan="2">Consider the history, geography, economic, and civics and government strands</td></tr>
<tr><td>X</td><td>Science and Technology</td><td colspan="2">Consider the inquiry, domains of science, technology and science, and technology and human affairs strands</td></tr>
<tr><td>X</td><td>Mathematics</td><td colspan="2">Consider the number sense, patterns, relations and functions, geometry and measurement, and statistics and probability strands</td></tr>
<tr><td>X</td><td>Other Curriculum Areas</td><td>Specify:</td><td>Health, Arts</td></tr>
<tr><td colspan="4">Whenever classroom demands and curriculum impinge on Leila's vulnerabilities in written output, focus, organization, or cognitive flexibility, she becomes dysregulated and disruptive in 3 out of 5 situations. Her reactivity then occludes her ability to consistently access curriculum and impacts the entire classroom environment. As a result, her social relationships are also impacted, socially isolating Leila.</td></tr>
</table>

The next section of PLEP A indicates what accommodations will be used in the classroom in order for Leila to access the curriculum (see Table 8.2). Now that we have the results of Leila's evaluation, we can utilize the lists of accommodations in previous chapters by selecting accommodations that match her assessment results and recommendations, classroom presentation, and interests. This includes addressing her attentional issues and consulting with an OT to provide a sensory diet, and support with graphomotor difficulties and organizational skills. In terms of functional domains, Leila requires support around her working memory, executive functioning skills, attentional capacity, handwriting, and organization of written projects.

The final section of PLEP A outlines the modifications, if any, that a student will need. Within this section, types of interventions may be briefly described as well as how progress will be assessed and measured (see Table 8.2).

As you can see, Leila does not require modified content. Her high cognitive scores reflect her ability to follow the Massachusetts CCSS without modifications. This indicates

TABLE 8.2 IEP Example: PLEP A Accommodations

*What type(s) of accommodation, **if any**, is necessary for the student to make effective progress?*
Step-by-step guidelines and procedures, color-coded Not required to take notes Provide review sheets in same format as the test Teach rehearsal strategies Access to multi-sensory lessons and study materials Pre-read textbook material before lectures Highlight key words in text Access to math formula sheets during testing Use of math manipulatives List of frequent writing/grammar errors to support editing Use of recorder for brainstorming Access to computer and organizational software Reduce workload Use of visual reminders for supplies and materials Use of timer to track time Provide structure and routine Frequently monitor performance and redirect as necessary Therapeutic behavioral modification plan Reduce distraction in the environment for assignments and tests Shorter duration on tasks Praise for completion of assignments Frequent breaks during class and testing Program in area of interest Provide visual cues for personal space Parents sign homework Consistent communication between home and school Highlight operation signs during calculation

TABLE 8.3 IEP Example: PLEP A Modifications

*What type(s) of accommodation, **if any**, is necessary for the student to make effective progress?*	
Check the necessary instructional modification(s) and describe how such modification(s) will be made.	
X Content:	Follow Mass. Common Core Curriculum
X Methodology/ Delivery of Instruction:	Multi-sensory approach to learning, access to therapeutic support, teach key concepts in short manageable chunks, direct instruction on organizational skills, explicit instruction on graphomotor skills, social skills group, individual occupational therapy, individual counseling
X Performance Criteria:	Quarterly IEP progress report, educational and psychological evaluation, consultation with specialists, extended time on assignments and tests, modified expectation of written responses and reports, opportunity for oral presentation, evaluation of work focuses on quality not quantity

that she is best suited to a mainstream classroom (or gifted classroom) at grade level. The methodology/delivery section focuses on providing additional supports and interventions that target Leila's vulnerabilities and make learning more accessible to her. Finally, the Performance Criteria section notes how her progress will be assessed. She will receive extra time on assignments and tests to accommodate her working memory difficulties and modifications to written assignments to accommodate her graphomotor difficulties. As a result of her attentional issues, she will not be required to do repetitive high-quantity work, but rather focus on quality.

Present Levels of Performance B

PLEP B is used to present ways in which Leila's difficulties impact other aspects of school education outside of accessing the curriculum. Note from the assessment results that Leila experiences difficulty with emotional and behavioral regulation, and that she desires social relationships but experiences difficulty navigating peer interactions. In PLEP B we can present information that will provide support for Leila in these areas, as they do impact her overall school experience and learning (see Table 8.4).

TABLE 8.4 IEP Example: PLEP B

Present Levels of Educational Performance *B: Other Educational Needs*
Check all that apply.
General Considerations
X__ Adapted physical education ____ Assistive tech devices/services X__ Behavior ___ Braille needs (blind/visually impaired) X__ Adapted physical education (deaf/hard of hearing students) ___ Communication

X____ Extra-curriculum activities _____ Language needs (LEP students) X___ Nonacademic activities X____ Social/emotional needs _____ Travel training ______ Skill development related to vocational preparation or experience X ___Other ____________________ Computer, Recess, Library, Lunch
Age-Specific Considerations
____ For children ages 3–5: participation in appropriate activities ____ For children ages 14+ (or younger if appropriate): student's course of study ____ For children ages 16 (or younger if appropriate) to 22: transition to post-school activities including community experiences, employment objectives, other post-school adult living and, if appropriate, daily living skills
Leila is an intellectually gifted young girl whose difficulties with graphomotor skills, executive functions, emotional and behavioral dysregulation, and extremely poor social skills have made school an overwhelming and unsuccessful experience. Because of her inadequate psychological and emotional resources, she has developed ineffective coping strategies that exacerbate relationships with peers and teachers. As a result, she has difficulty navigating social situations, negotiating disagreements, and developing age-appropriate social skills. This results in compounding anxiety, which impacts her ability to access curriculum.

TABLE 8.5 IEP Example: PLEP B Accommodations

*What type(s) of accommodation, **if any**, is necessary for the student to make effective progress?*
Access to therapeutic staff Quiet space for breaks Close monitoring during social interaction, provide scaffolding Provide scripts for social situations Preview new situations and expectations Designated individual within school environment for processing social situations Create scenarios in which the student will experience success Clear frequent communication between home and school Planned ignoring for selected behaviors Self-monitoring checklist Choices within limits Positive intervention plan Consistency across environments Building relationships with adults Reflect and process after behavioral incidents Modification of workload Allow opportunities for movement breaks Model appropriate responses to social situations Target perspective-taking skills Private feedback on assignments Advance notice on assignments Immediately praise appropriate behavior Specify rewards for following rules and consequences for disobeying rules

TABLE 8.6 IEP Example: PLEP B Modifications

*What type(s) of specifically designed instruction, **if any**, is necessary for the student to make effective progress?*	
Check the necessary instructional modification(s) and describe how such modification(s) will be made.	
X Content:	Simplified and modified, teach key concepts in manageable chunks, coping strategies, organizational skills, graphomotor skills, managing emotion, identifying triggers, explicitly teach social skills and rules, teach and practice active listening
X Methodology/ Delivery of Instruction:	Teach in manageable chunks, individual counseling, social skills group, individual occupational therapy, modeling and roleplaying, books, behavior or emotions charts/tools geared toward regulation
X Performance Criteria:	Quarterly IEP progress report, consultation with specialists, progress toward IEP goals, information from therapeutic charts, allow extra time on assessments and graded projects

Accommodations in PLEP B are designed to address Leila's needs in this area and can be pulled from the previous chapters on social/emotional/behavioral skills and executive functioning skills (see Table 8.5).

The final section of PLEP B addresses specific interventions, delivery methods, and modifications that can support Leila (see Table 8.6). Note that in the Performance Criteria section, extra time for assessments and graded projects is included despite the social/emotional nature of the PLEP B. This is because social/emotional regulation is tied to academic performance and this should be reflected in all aspects of the IEP.

Writing Measurable Goals

Given the assessment results and diagnoses related to Leila's presentation, her IEP goals should reflect her academic and social/emotional needs. There should be goals related to organization, social/emotional regulation, graphomotor development (written in consultation with an occupational therapist), and writing. We will focus on the social/emotional goals, as these can often be the most difficult to make measurable and concrete.

TABLE 8.7 IEP Example: Current Performance Level

Current Performance Levels/Measurable Annual Goals		
Goal #		Specific Goal Focus: Emotional/Behavioral
Current Performance Level: What can the student currently do?		
Leila is a bright and thoughtful student who desires friendship and academic success. However, her difficulties with executive functions, emotional regulation, graphomotor skills, and attentional issues often impede her ability to access the curriculum, resulting in low self-esteem, frustration, dysregulation, and disruptive behavior. She currently uses inappropriate coping mechanisms to manage anxiety around her difficulties – such as self-inflated importance, pointing out the faults of others, and arguing with teachers and peers. These maladaptive coping mechanisms further isolate Leila, despite her desire for friendship and success. She can be humorous, caring, and generous, especially when engaged in preferred activities.		

Under the current performance level, results of the evaluation and teacher observation can be used to describe Leila's current abilities (see Table 8.7).

The description of her current performance points out some strengths and her desire for friendships. It also discusses her vulnerabilities and how they manifest behaviorally in the classroom. It acknowledges that her behavioral responses and coping mechanisms are rooted in underlying learning disabilities. The language in the goal and measured benchmarks focuses on providing Leila with new coping skills so that she can access her strengths more easily.

Note that the goal and benchmarks indicate the frequency in which she engages in a specific activity or behavior and an attainable goal to work toward (see Table 8.8).

TABLE 8.8 IEP Example: Measurable Goals and Benchmarks

Measurable Annual Goal: What challenging, yet attainable, goal can we expect the student to meet by the end of this IEP period? How will we know that the student has reached this goal?
Leila will develop and utilize strategies for regulating her behavior and emotions, with decreasing support in 3 out of 5 trials.
Benchmark/Objectives: What will the student need to do to complete this goal?
1) Leila will utilize a feelings chart throughout the day to monitor her mood, with decreasing support in 3 out of 5 trials. 2) Leila will refrain from making negative comments during non-preferred activities and receive positive reinforcement from a therapeutic behavioral plan in 3 out of 5 trials. 3) Leila will accurately label her emotions, with therapeutic support, utilizing a feelings grid, in 3 out of 5 trials. 4) Leila will appropriately ask for help when confused, frustrated or bored, with decreasing support in 3 out of 5 trials.

–9–

Working with the Family

As a child grows and participates in more environments outside of the home, these environments have the potential to become part of the holding environment (Hyman, 2012). Just as one attempts to create a holding environment through a relationship established between a teacher/specialist and child, it is equally important to establish a relationship between a teacher/specialist and parents. Doing so creates a holding environment that encompasses school and home. Establishing an alliance with parents is a crucial part of this process. Integrating the results of a neuropsychological evaluation into the school day is also part of creating and maintaining the holding environment. Any attempt to integrate findings from testing and sustain successful interventions that will evolve over time must include a coordinated approach between home and school.

Research supports the need for schools and families to work together to support students at all grades. Northey et al. (2003) found that family based interventions were superior to individual interventions for children with externalizing disorders when parents were also experiencing emotional difficulties. In another study, Hogue and Dauber (2006) found that family focused therapy predicted a decrease in children's internalizing and externalizing symptoms and had a positive impact on family conflict. Family involvement also impacts a child's academic success (Vennum & Vennum, 2013). One of the best ways to involve parents (or guardians) is to institute and maintain effective communication. In order to ensure that communication is successful, a mutual understanding of how communication is to be established, how to sustain communication and an appreciation of how boundaries will be respected is critical.

One of the mantras that have become part of our litany over the years at CTDS is that "home and school work together." This is often said as a way of reassuring a child that their worlds are making the effort to provide him/her with an experience that is consistent and somewhat predictable. In this manner, the child feels seen, held, and cared for within important relationships and therefore feels safe to explore and learn. An education cannot proceed when a child feels the tension between teachers and parents who maintain significantly different perspectives on what a child needs or what is expected of him/her. That does not mean that school personnel and parents will always immediately agree on what course to take. It does mean, however, that there must be an established vehicle with which differences can be understood, respected, and worked through to present a unified front to the child.

Within the context of integrating interventions recommended by a neuropsychological evaluation, it is important to establish from the beginning an explicit understanding of how services and approaches will be coordinated between home and school. Whenever an evaluation is completed by a school or a private evaluation is presented to the school by the parents, the school is responsible for convening a team meeting within 10 school days. At this meeting, as services are determined, there should be an in-depth discussion of how these interventions will be coordinated between home and school. This requires considerable sensitivity on the part of school personnel in an effort to respect both the strengths and vulnerabilities which parents bring to this discussion, as well as the strengths and vulnerabilities inherent within the rest of the team. Presenting a plan that has been generated by all involved in a clear, straightforward, and realistic manner will establish a foundation for future communication. Depending on the level of need, as determined by an evaluation as well as the experiences of school personnel and parents, any combination of the following modes of communication could be employed:

- *Communication Book* – This is used to facilitate daily communication and travels back and forth between home and school every morning and afternoon. Parents are encouraged to write in the book, detailing any significant events that occurred at home. These could include any observations about homework (e.g., math was difficult, reading went well, refusal to write an assignment), difficulty getting to sleep, an upsetting event during play with a friend, a parent's illness or trip away from home, a change in medication, or a trip to the doctor. This way the teacher will have some sense of what may be impacting the child's ability to engage in school, provide information with which to acknowledge any difficulty the child may be having, and help contain any worries. Similarly, information provided by the teacher to the parent will alert parents to any events that occurred during the school day that may impact the child's ability to do homework, tolerate frustration, or manage the demands of the home environment, or affect their willingness to return to school. This should also include any successes the child has had so that the information appears balanced, providing a sense of the child's areas of strength and areas in which they continue to struggle. When the child is included in the sharing of this information, it can reinforce the message that home and school are working together. The information provided by the teacher should be factual, outlining details that are significant, and should not include interpretation beyond the facts or appear judgmental.
- *Email* – Many teachers are now using email to communicate with parents. Certain precautions must be considered, however, if this is to be a significant form of interaction. Most importantly, the email system being used must be HIPPA (Health Insurance Portability and Accountability Act) compliant. This ensures that any information transmitted via email is secure and that an individual's privacy is respected and safe from any unauthorized viewing. If the system is not HIPPA compliant, then there should not be any sharing of clinically sensitive information or any information with which the parent is not comfortable potentially being made public.
- *Phone communication* – Direct verbal communication on a regular basis can supplement the daily written communication. We have found that a weekly phone call can provide an opportunity to discuss information in more detail as well as an opportunity

to engage in more of a give-and-take dialogue. Communication of this sort can also be used to clarify information in the book or clear up any miscommunications.

- *Regular face-to-face meetings* – This form of communication is often the best means toward developing a close working relationship between parents and school personnel. Meetings held, for example, on a monthly basis serve to further reinforce the sense that there is a group of concerned and committed adults who are working together to provide the holding that the child requires. This, in turn, helps parents feel that they too are being held by others who understand their particular struggle and who support their efforts.
- *Community Events* – In addition to individualized means of communication, holding annual community events is another means for developing rapport and supporting families. Annual Back to School nights allow family members to view a child's classroom with the child. Holding annual family focused events (BBQs/picnics, science fairs, fundraisers, and alumni events) continues to provide a sense of a larger community that can include all family members (siblings, grandparents, etc.), fostering engagement on multiple levels. The type of family work described above is clearly intensive and time-consuming. It requires an awareness of how a particular family's set of characteristics may trigger thoughts and feelings that can be challenging. It is important to recognize that any approach to family work of this sort demands that school personnel adopt the perspective that the parents are the experts regarding their child and that, barring extreme circumstances, they have the best interest of the child in mind. Parents of a child with special needs are on a journey they did not imagine. Their idea of their child moving through a "normal" educational process has been detoured and many parents are at a loss as to how to proceed. As educational specialists, teachers, counselors, and other personnel, we are in a unique position to provide a roadmap that is guided by information obtained from careful and thorough evaluation and ongoing observation. To be successful, this new route must be planned, tried, updated, and revised as many times as necessary, and always in collaboration with all those involved.

Conclusion

Having worked as teachers of children with significant special needs and now serving as professionals who assess children and consult to school systems that attempt to accommodate and support those children, we are particularly sympathetic to the conundrum that teachers and specialists face. We hope this manual serves to assist you in your efforts to interpret results from neuropsychological and psychological assessments and implement those findings. Most importantly, we are hopeful that the provision of an easily accessed and practical means to translate and apply those results facilitates the most crucial component of the process: the development of holding environments in which understanding, compassion, and relationships serve as the foundation for learning.

References

Adolph, K. E., Eppler, M. A., & Gibson, E. J. (1993). Crawling versus walking infants' perception of affordances for locomotion over sloping surfaces. *Child Development*, *64*(4), 1158–1174.

Ainsworth, M. D. S., Blear, M. C., Waters, E., & Wall, S. (1978). *Patterns of attachment: A psychological study of the strange situation*. Hillsdale, NJ: Erlbaum.

Alberto, P., Heflin, L. J., & Andrews, D. (2002). Use of the timeout ribbon procedure during community-based instruction. *Behavior Modification*, *26*, 297–311.

Alberts, C. A., & Feeney-Kettler, K. A. (2014). *Universal screening in educational settings: Evidence-based decision making for schools*. New York, NY: American Psychological Association.

Ali, A., Aziz, Z., & Majzub, R. (2011). Teaching and learning reading through play. *World Applied Sciences Journal (Learning Innovation and Intervention for Diverse Learners)*, *14*, 15–20.

Alloway, T. P., & Passolunghi, M. C. (2011). The relationship between working memory, IQ and mathematical skills in children. *Learning and Individual Differences*, *21*(1), 133–137.

Anderson, P. (2002). Assessment and development of executive function (EF) during childhood. *Child Neuropsychology*, *8*(2), 1–82.

Anderson, S. W. (2002). Visuoperceptual impairments. In P. J. Eslinger (Ed.), *Neuropsychological interventions: Clinical research and practice*. New York, NY: The Guildford Press.

Autin, F., & Croizet, J. C. (2012). Improving working memory efficiency by reframing metacognitive interpretation of task difficulty. *Journal of Experimental Psychology: General*, *141*(4), 610–618.

Baker, J. A. (2006). Contributions of teacher–child relationships to positive school adjustment during elementary school. *Journal of School Psychology*, *44*, 211– 229.

Baker, J. A., Grant, S., & Morlock, L. (2008). The teacher–student relationship as a developmental context for children with internalizing or externalizing behavior problems. *School Psychology Quarterly*, *23*, 3–15.

Bakermans-Kranenburg, M. J., van Ijzendoorn, M. H., & Juffer, F. (2003). Less is more: Meta-analyses of sensitivity and attachment interventions in early childhood. *Psychological Bulletin*, *129*, 195–215.

Baron-Cohen, S. (2008). Autism in 100 words. *The British Journal of Psychiatry*, *193*, 321.

Barrett, L. F., & Bar, M. (2009). See it with feeling: Affective predictions during object perception. *Philosophical Transactions of the Royal Society of London: B Biological Sciences*, *364*, 1325–1334.

Bayley, N. (2006). *Bayley scales of infant and toddler development* (3rd ed). San Antonio, TX: Harcourt Assessment.

Beery, K. E., Buktenica, N. A., & Beery, N. (2010). *The Beery–Buktenica developmental test of visual-motor integration* (6th ed.). San Antonio, TX: Pearson.

Benner, G. J., Nelson, J. R., & Epstein, M. H. (2002). Language skills of children with EDB: A literature review. *Journal of Emotional and Behavioral Disorders, 10*(1), 43–56.
Berninger, V., & Graham, S. (1998). Language by hand: A synthesis of a decade of research on handwriting. *Handwriting Review, 12*, 11–25.
Berry, D., & O'Connor, E. (2010). Behavioral risk, teacher–child relationships, and social skill development across middle childhood: A child-by-environment analysis of change. *Journal of Applied Developmental Psychology, 31*, 1–14.
Best, J. R., & Miller, P. H. (2010). A developmental perspective on executive function. *Child Development, 81*(6), 1641–1660. http://doi.org/10.1111/j.1467-8624.2010.01499.x.
Biederman, J., Newcorn, J., & Sprich, S. (1991). Comorbidity of attention deficit hyperactivity disorder with conduct, depressive, anxiety and other disorders. *American Journal of Psychiatry, 148*, 546–577.
Bierman, K. L., Nix, R. L., Greenberg, M. T., Blair, C., & Domitrovich, C. E. (2008). Executive functions and school readiness intervention: Impact, moderation, and mediation in the Head Start REDI program. *Development and Psychopathology, 20*, 821–843.
Birney, D. P., & Sternberg, R. J. (2011). The development of cognitive abilities. In M. H. Bornstein & M. E. Lamb (Eds.), *Developmental science: An advanced textbook* (6th ed.) (pp. 353–388). New York, NY: Psychology Press.
Bornstein, M. H. (2006). Hue categorization and color naming: Physics to sensation to perception. In N. J. Pitchford & C. P. Biggam (Eds.), *Progress in colour studies, Vol. II. Psychological aspects* (pp. 35–68). Amsterdam/Philadelphia, PA: John Benjamins.
Bornstein, M. H. (2007). Hue categorization and color naming: Cognition to language to culture. In R. E. MacLaury, G. V. Paramei, & D. Dedrick (Eds.), *Anthropology of color: Interdisciplinary multilevel modeling* (pp. 3–27). Amsterdam/Philadelphia, PA: John Benjamins.
Bornstein, M. H., Arterberry, M. E., & Mash, C. (2011). Perceptual development. In M. H. Bornstein & M. E. Lamb (Eds.), *Developmental science: An advanced textbook* (6th ed.). New York, NY: Taylor and Francis Group.
Bornstein, M. H., Ferdinandsen, K., & Gross, C. G. (1981). Perception of symmetry in infancy. *Developmental Psychology, 17*, 82–86.
Bornstein, M. H., Kessen, W., & Weiskopf, S. (1976). The categories of hue in infancy. *Science, 191*, 201–202.
Bowlby, J. (1982). *Development in infancy* (2nd ed.). New York, NY: W. H. Freeman.
Bowlby, J. (1988). *A secure base: Parent-child attachment and healthy human development.* New York, NY: Basic Books.
Braaten, E., & Willoughby, B. (2014). *Bright kids who can't keep up: Help your child overcome slow processing speed and succeed in a fast-paced world.* New York, NY: Guilford Publications.
Brandon, A., Salkind, S., Golnikoff, R. M., & Hirsh-Pasek, K. (2006). Language development. In G. Bear & K. Minke (Eds.), *Children's needs: Development, prevention and intervention* (pp. 499–514). Bethesda, MD: National Association of School Psychologists.
Briesch, A. M., & Chafouleas, S. M. (2009). Review and analysis of literature on self-management interventions to promote appropriate classroom behavior (1988–2008). *School Psychology Quarterly, 24*, 106–118.
Britzman, D. P. (2009). *The very thought of education: Psychoanalysis and the impossible professions.* Albany, NY: Sate University Press of New York Press.
Britzman, D. P., & Dippo, D. (2000). On the future of awful thoughts in education. *Teaching Education, 11*(1), 31–37.

Bronfenbrenner, U., & Evans, G. W. (2000). Developmental science in the 21st century: Emerging questions, theoretical models, research designs and empirical findings. *Social Development, 9*(1), 115–125.

Brown, S., & Vaughan, C. (2009). *Play: How it shapes the brain, opens the imagination and invigorates the soul.* New York, NY: Penguin Group.

Bryant, D. P., Pfannenstiel, K. H., Bryant, B. R., Hunt, J., & Shin, M. (2014). Selecting and tailoring interventions for students with mathematics difficulties. In J. T. Mascolo, V. C. Alfonos, & D. P. Flanagan (Eds.), *Essentials of planning, selecting and tailoring interventions for unique learners.* Hoboken, NJ: John Wiley & Sons.

Bull, R., & Espy, K. A. (2006). Working memory, executive functioning and children's mathematics. In S. J. Pickering (Ed.), *Working memory and education.* Burlington, MA: Elsevier.

Bull, R., & Johnston, R. S. (1997). Children's arithmetical difficulties: Contributions from processing speed, item identification, and short-term memory. *Journal of Experimental Child Psychology, 65,* 1–24.

Bundy, A., Cordier, R., & Lincoln, M. (2014). Eighteen-month follow-up of play-based intervention to improve the social play skills of children with attention deficit hyperactivity disorder. *Australian Occupational Therapy Journal, 61,* 299–307.

Bus, A. G., & van Ijzendoorn, M. H. (1988). Mother–child interactions, attachment, and emergent literacy: A cross-sectional study. *Child Development, 59,* 1262–1272.

Buyse, E., Verschueren, K., Doumen, S., Van Damme, J., & Maes, F. (2008). Classroom problem behavior and teacher–child relationships in kindergarten: The moderating role of classroom climate. *Journal of School Psychology, 46,* 367–391.

Cain, K. (2006). Children's reading comprehension: The role of working memory in normal and impaired development. In S. J. Pickering (Ed.), *Working memory and education.* Burlington, MA: Elsevier.

Canas, J. J., Quesada, J. F., Antoli, A., & Fajardo, I. (2003). Cognitive flexibility and adaptability to environmental changes in dynamic complex problem-solving tasks. *Ergonomics, 46,* 482–501.

Canter, L. (2001). *Assertive discipline: Positive behavior management for today's classroom.* Canter & Associates, vi, 234.

Carey, S., Diamond, R., & Woods, B. (1980). Development of face recognition: A maturational component. *Developmental Psychology, 16,* 257–269.

Carlson, A. G., Rowe, E., & Curby, T. W. (2013). Disentangling fine motor skills' relations to academic achievement: The relative contributions of visual-spatial integration and visual-motor coordination. *Journal of Genetic Psychology, 174*(5), 514–533.

Carlson, S. M., Claxton, L. J., & Moses, L. J. (2015). The relation between executive function and theory of mind is more than skin deep. *Journal of Cognition and Development, 16*(1), 186–197.

Carlson, S. M., White, R. E., & Davis-Unger, A. C. (2014). Evidence for a relation between executive function and pretense representation in preschool children. *Cognitive Development, 29,* 315–334.

Carter, R. (2009). *The human brain book.* New York, NY: DK Publishing.

Carty, M. (2000). *Surviving and thriving: Making classroom organization work for you and your students.* Markham, CA: Pembroke Publishers.

Carver, L. J. (2013). Cognitive neuroscience of emotion and memory development. In P. J. Bauer and R. Fivush (Eds.), *The Wiley handbook on the development of children's memory, Vol. I/II.* Chichester: John Wiley & Sons.

Casey, B. M., Anders, N., Schindler, H., Kersh, J. E., Samper, A., & Copley, J. (2008). The development of spatial skills through interventions involving block building activities. *Cognition and Instruction, 26,* 269–309.

Casey, B. M., Pezaris, E. E., & Bassi, J. (2012). Adolescent boys' and girls' block constructions differ in structural balance: A block-building characteristic related to math achievement. *Learning and Individual Differences*, *22*(1), 25–36.
Cattell, R. B. (1971). *Abilities: Their structure, growth and action*. Boston, MA: Houghton Mifflin.
Center on the Developing Child at Harvard University (2014). *Enhancing and practicing executive function skills with children from infancy to adolescence*. Retrieved from www.developingchild.harvard.edu.
Cherry, J. (n.d.). Dysgraphia & math: Difficulties & accommodations. Retrieved from http://study.com/academy/lesson/dysgraphia-math-difficulties-accommodations.html.
Cleary, M. J., & Scott, A. J. (2011). Developments in clinical neuropsychology: Implications for school psychological services. *Journal of School Health*, *81*(1), 1–7.
Coie, J. D., Terry, R., Lenox, K., & Lockman, J. (1995). Childhood peer rejection and aggression as predictors of stable patterns of adolescent disorder. *Development and Psychology*, *7*, 697–713.
Cole, P., Duncan, L. G., & Blaye, A. (2014). Cognitive flexibility predicts early reading skills. *Frontiers in Psychology*, *5*, 1–8.
College Committee on Disability Issues (2008). *LD resource guide: Accommodations, learning strategies, assertive technology and universal design for instruction*. Retrieved from www.disabilityissues.ca/english/Link_docs/LDResour.pdf.
Colvin, G. (1993). *Managing the cycle of acting-out behavior*. Eugene, OR: Behavior Associates.
Colvin, G. (1997). *The effective elementary classroom*. Longmont, CO: Spoors West Publishing.
Cooper, J. O., Heron, T. E., & Heward, W. L. (2007). *Applied behavioral analysis* (2nd ed.). Upper Saddle River, NJ: Pearson/Prentice Hall.
Cook, J. (2006). *My mouth is a volcano!* Chattanooga, TN: National Center of Youth Issues.
Cowan, N. (2008). What are the differences between long-term, short-term, and working memory? *Progress in Brain Research*, *169*, 323–338.
Crone, D. A., & Horner, R. H. (2003). *Building positive behavior support systems in schools: Functional behavioral assessment*. New York, NY: Guildford.
Crundwell, R. M., & Killu, K. (2007). Accommodating students with depression in the classroom. *Teaching Exceptional Children*, 40.
Cunningham, P. M., & Allington, R. L. (1994). *Classrooms that work: They can all read and write*. New York, NY: HarperCollins.
Davis, A., & Bamford, G. (1995). The effect of imagery on young children's ability to solve simple arithmetic. *Education Section Review*, *19*, 61–68.
Davis, E. E., Pitchford, N. J., & Limback, E. (2011). The interrelation between cognitive and motor development in typically developing children aged 4–11 years is underpinned by visual processing and fine manual control. *British Journal of Psychology*, *102*, 569–584.
Dawson, P., & Guare, R. (2010). *Executive skills in children and adolescents: A practical guide to assessment and intervention* (2nd ed.). New York, NY: Guilford Press.
Dehaene, S. (2009). *Reading and the brain*. New York, NY: Penguin Group.
Dehn, M. J. (2011). *Working memory and academic learning: Assessment and intervention*. Hoboken, NJ: John Wiley & Sons.
Dehn, M. J. (2012). *Children's psychological process scale*. Onalaska, WI: Schoolhouse Educational Services.

Dehn, M. J. (2014). Interventions for students with memory difficulties. In J. T. Mascolo, V. C. Alfonso, & D. P. Flanagan (Eds.), *Essentials of planning, selecting and tailoring interventions for unique learners*. Hoboken, NJ: John Wiley & Sons.
Denham, S. A., Bassett, H. H., Mincic, M. M., Kalb, S. C., Way, E., Wyatt, T., & Segal, Y. (2012). Social-emotional learning profiles of preschoolers' early school success: A person-centered approach. *Learning and Individual Differences*, *22*, 178–189.
Denham, S. A., Bassett, H. H., Zinsser, K., & Wyatt, T. M. (2014). How preschoolers' social-emotional learning predicts their early school success: Developing theory-promoting, competency-based assessments. *Infant and Child Development*, *23*, 426–454.
Desote, A., & De Weerdt, F. (2013). Can executive function help to understand children with mathematical learning disorders and to improve instruction? *Learning Disabilities: A Contemporary Journal*, *11*(2), 27–39.
Deuel, R. K. (1994). Developmental dysgraphia and motor skills disorders. *Journal of Child Neurology*, *10*, 6–8.
Deutsch, D., Henthorn, T., & Dolson, M. (2004). Speech patterns heard early in life influence later perception of the tritone paradox. *Music Perception*, *21*, 357–372.
Diamond, R., Carey, S., & Back, K. J. (1983). Genetic influences on the development of spatial skills during adolescence. *Cognition*, *13*, 167–185.
Droit-Volet, S., & Zelanti, P. S. (2013). Development of time sensitivity and information processing speed. *PLoS ONE*, *8*(8), 1–9.
Dunlap, L. K., & Dunlap, G. (1989). A self-monitoring package for teaching subtraction with regrouping to students with learning disabilities. *Journal of Applied Behavior Analysis*, *229*, 309–314.
Ehlers, A., & Clark, D. M. (2000). A cognitive model of post-traumatic stress disorder. *Behavior Research and Therapy*, *38*, 319–345.
Elkind, D. (2007). *The power of play*. Philadelphia, PA: Da Capo Press.
Elliot, C. D. (2007). *Differential ability scales* (2nd ed.). San Antonio, TX: Harcourt Assessment.
Emmer, E. T., Evertson, C. M., & Anderson, L. D. (1980). Effective management at the beginning of the school year. *Elementary School Journal*, *80*, 219–231.
Fanti, K. A., & Henrich, C. C. (2010). Trajectories of pure and co-occurring internalizing and externalizing problems from age 2 to age 12: Findings from the National Institute of Child Health and Human Development Study of Early Child Care. *Developmental Psychology*, *46*(5), 1159–1175.
Fantuzzo, J. W., Rohrbeck, C. A., & Azar, S. T. (1987). A component analysis of behavioral self-management interventions with elementary school students. *Child and Family Behavior Therapy*, *9*, 33–43.
Feder, K. P., & Majnemer, A. (2007). Handwriting development, competency and intervention. *Developmental Medicine and Child Neurology*, *49*, 312–317.
Ferrer, E., Whitaker, K. J., Steele, J. S., Green, C. T., Wendelken, C., & Bunge, S. A. (2013). White matter maturation supports the development of reasoning ability through its influence on processing speed. *Developmental Science*, *16*(6), 941–951.
Finnegan, R. A., Hodges, E. E., & Perry, D. G. (1996). Preoccupied and avoidant coping during middle childhood. *Child Development*, *67*(4), 1318–1328.
First Years (2011). Retrieved from http://firstyears.org/miles/chart.htm.
Fitzgerald, J., & Shanahan, T. (2000). Reading and writing relations and their development. *Educational Psychologist*, *35*(1), 39–50.
Flanagan, D. P., Ortiz, S. O., Alfonso, V. C., & Mascolo, J. T. (2002). *The achievement test desk reference: Comprehensive assessment and learning disabilities*. Boston, MA: Allyn & Bacon.

Forrest, B. (2007). Diagnosing and treating right hemisphere disorders. In S. J. Hunter & J. Donders (Eds.), *Pediatric neuropsychological intervention* (pp. 175–192). Cambridge: Cambridge University Press.

Franklin, A., & Davies, I. R. L. (2004). New evidence for infant colour categories. *British Journal of Developmental Psychology*, *22*, 349–377.

Frith, U. (1985). Beneath the surface of developmental dyslexia. *Surface Dyslexia*, *32*, 301–330.

Frye, D., Baroody, A. J., Burchinal, M., Carver, S. M., Jordan, N. C., & McDowell, J. (2013). *Teaching math to young children: A practice guide* (NCEE 2014–4005). Washington, DC: National Center for Education Evaluation and Regional Assistance (NCEE), Institute of Education Sciences, U. S. Department of Education. Retrieved from http://whatworks.ed.gov.

Fuchs, L. S., Compton, D. L., Fuchs, D., Paulsen, K., & Bryant, B. R. (2005). Responsiveness to intervention: Preventing and identifying mathematics disability. *Teaching Exceptional Children*, *37*(4), 60–63.

Fujiki, M., Brinton, B., Hart, C. H., & Fitzgerald, A. H. (1999). Peer acceptance and friendship in children with specific language impairment. *Topics in Language Disorders*, *19*(2), 34–48.

Gable, R. A., Park, K. L., & Scott, T. M. (2014). Functional behavioral assessment and students at risk for or with emotional disabilities: Current issues and considerations. *Education & Treatment of Children*, *37*(1), 111–135.

Gallahue, D. L., & Ozmun, J. C. (2002). *Understanding motor development*. Boston, MA: McGraw-Hill.

Garner, P. W., & Lemerise, E. A. (2007). The roles of behavior adjustment and conceptions of peers and emotions in preschool children's peer victimization. *Development and Psychopathology*, *19*, 57–71.

Garner, P. W., & Waajid, B. (2008). The associations of emotion knowledge and teacher–child relationship to preschool children's school-related developmental competence. *Journal of Applied Development Psychology*, *29*(2), 89–100.

Garnett, K. (1998). Math learning disabilities. LD Online. Retrieved from www.ldonline.org/article/ Math_Learning_Disabilities?theme=print.

Gathercole, S. E., Lamont, E., & Alloway, T. P. (2006). Working memory in the classroom. In S. J. Pickering (Ed.), *Working memory and education*. Burlington, MA: Elsevier.

Gazelle, H. (2006). Class climate moderates peer relations and emotional adjustment in children with an early history of anxious solitude: A child X environment model. *Developmental Psychology*, *42*, 1179–1192.

Geary, D. C. (1994). Developing arithmetical skills. In *Children's mathematical development: Research and practical applications* (pp. 37–93). Washington, DC: American Psychological Association.

Geary, D. C. (2004). Mathematics and learning disabilities. *Journal of Learning Disabilities*, *37*, 4–15.

Geary, D. C., Hoard, M. K., Byrd-Craven, J., Nugent, L., & Numtee, C. (2007). Cognitive mechanisms underlying achievement deficits in children with mathematical learning disability. *Child Development*, *33*, 277–299.

Geddes, H. (2006). *Attachment in the classroom*. London: Worth Publishing.

Gil, E. (2006). *Helping abused and traumatized children*. New York, NY: The Guildford Press.

Gilmore, K. (2002). Diagnosis, dynamics, and development: Considerations in the psychoanalytic assessment of children with AD/HD. *A Topical Journal for Mental Health Professionals*, *3*, 372–390.

Glass, K. L., Guli, L. A., & Segmund-Clickman, M. (2000). Social competence intervention program: A pilot study for the develop of social competence. *Journal of Psychotherapy in Independent Practice, Special Issue, Social Competence and Developmental Disorders, 1*, 21–33.

Gordon, T., & Burch, N. (1974). *T. E. T., Teacher effectiveness training*. New York, NY: P. H. Wyden.

Grafen, J., Kohn, J., Wyschkon, A., & Esser, G. (2015). Internalizing problems in children and adolescents with math disability. *Zeitschrift fur Psychologie, 223*(2), 93–101.

Graham, S. (1990). The roles of production factors in learning disabled students' compositions. *Journal of Educational Psychology, 82*, 781–791.

Graham, S., & Weintraub, N. (1996). A review of handwriting research: Progress and prospects from 1980–1994. *Educational Psychology Review, 8*, 7–86.

Graziano, P. A., Reavis, R. D., Keane, S. P., & Calkins, S. D. (2007). The role of emotion regulation in children's early academic success. *Journal of School Psychology, 45*, 3–19.

Greenham, S. L. (1999). Learning disabilities and psychosocial adjustment: A critical review. *Child Neuropsychology, 5*, 171–196.

Guanella, F. (1934). Block building activities of young children. *Archives of Psychology (Columbia University), 174*, 92.

Guli, L. A. (2005). The effect of creative drama-based intervention for children with deficits in social perception. *Dissertation Abstracts International Section A: Humanities and Social Sciences, 65*, 3690.

Haith, M. M. (2004). Progress and standardization in eye movement work with human infants. *Infancy, 6*, 257–265.

Hamre, B. K., & Pianta, R. C. (2001). Early teacher–child relationships and the trajectory of children's school outcomes through eighth grade. *Child Development, 72*, 625–638.

Han, M., Moore, N., Vukelich, C., & Buell, M. (2010). Does play make a difference? How play intervention affects the vocabulary learning of at-risk preschoolers. *American Journal of Play, 3*(1), 82–105.

Harrington, R., & Clark, A. (1998). Prevention and early intervention for depression in adolescence and early adult life. *European Archives of Psychiatry and Clinical Neuroscience, 248*, 32–45.

Harris, J. R. (1996). Verbal rehearsal and memory in children with closed head injury: A quantitative and qualitative analysis. *Journal of Communication Disorders, 29*, 79–93.

Hill, E. (2004). Evaluating the theory of executive dysfunction in autism. *Developmental Review, 24*, 189–233.

Hill, J. W., & Coufal, K. L. (2005). Emotional/behavioral disorders: A retrospective examination of social skills, linguistics, and student outcomes. *Educational Leadership Faculty Publications*. Paper 3. Omaha, NE: University of Nebraska at Omaha.

Hinz, L. D. (2009). *Expressive therapies continuum: A framework for using art in therapy*. New York, NT: Routledge Publishing.

Hogue, A., & Dauber, S. (2006). Treatment techniques and outcomes in multidimensional family therapy for adolescent behavior problems. *Journal of Family Psychology, 20*, 535–543.

Holmes-Bernstein, J., & Weiler, M. D. (2000). Pediatric neuropsychological assessment examined. In G. Goldstein & M. Hersen (Eds.), *Handbook of psychological assessment* (3rd ed.). Kidlington, Oxford: Elsevier Science.

Hoover, J. J., Baca, L., Wexler-Lover, E., & Saenz, L. (2008). Implementation of response to intervention (RTI): Research summary. Special education leadership and quarterly initiative. Boulder, CO: BUENO Center for Multicultural Education, University of Colorado Boulder.

Horn, J. L. (1988). Thinking about human abilities. In R. J. Sternberg (Ed.), *The encyclopedia of human intelligence, Vol. 1* (pp. 443–451). New York, NY: Macmillan.
Huberty, T. (2008). Best practices in school-based interventions for anxiety and depression. In A. Thomas & Grimes, J. (Eds.), *Best practices in school psychology V* (pp. 1473–1486). Bethesda, MD: National Association of School Psychologists.
Huntington, D. D., & Bender, W. N. (1993). Adolescents with learning disabilities at risk? Emotional well-being, depression, suicide. *Journal of Learning Disabilities, 26*, 159–166.
Hyman, S. (2012). The school as a holding environment. *Journal of Infant, Child and Adolescent Psychotherapy, 11*(3), 205–216.
Hymel, S., Rubin, K. H., Rowden, L., & LeMare, L. (1990). Children's peer relationships: Longitudinal prediction of internalizing and externalizing problems from middle to late childhood. *Child Development, 61*, 2004–2021.
Jennings, J. L., & DiPrete, T. A. (2010). Teacher effects on social and behavioral skills in early elementary school. *Sociology of Education, 83*, 135–159.
Jennings, S. (2011). *Healthy attachments and neuro-dramatic play.* Philadelphia, PA: Jessica Kingsley Publishers.
Johnson, M. H., & Morton, J. (1991). *Biology and cognitive development.* Oxford: Blackwell.
Johnson, J. E., Christie, J. F., & Wardle, F. (2005). *Play, development and early education.* New York, NY: Pearson.
Jolivette, K., Wehby, J. H., & Hirsch, L. (1999). Academic strategy identification for students exhibiting inappropriate classroom behaviors. *Behavioral Disorders, 42*, 210–221.
Jones, D., & Christensen, C. A. (1999). Relationship between automaticity in handwriting and student's ability to generate written text. *Journal of Educational Psychology, 91*, 44–49.
Jones, K., & Day, J. (1996). Cognitive similarities between academically and socially gifted students. *Roper Review: A Journal on Gifted Education, 18*(4), 270–273.
Kaduson, H., & Schaefer, C. (Eds.) (1997). *101 favorite play therapy techniques.* Northvale, NJ: Jason Aronson.
Kail, R. (1991). Developmental change in speed of processing during childhood and adolescence. *Psychological Bulletin, 109*, 490–501.
Kail, R., & Ferrer, E. (2007). Processing speed in childhood and adolescence: Longitudinal models for examining developmental change. *Child Development, 78*(6), 1760–1770.
Kail, R. V., McBride-Chang, C., Ferrer, E., Cho, J., & Shu, H. (2013). Cultural differences in the development of processing speed. *Developmental Science, 16*(3), 476–483.
Kamii, C., Miyakawa, Y., & Kato, Y. (2004). The development of logico-mathematical knowledge in a block-building activity at ages 1–4. *Journal of Research in Childhood Education, 19*(1), 44–57.
Kataoka, S., Langley, A., Wong, M., Bawega, S., & Stein, B. (2012). Responding to students with PTSD in schools. *Child and Adolescent Psychiatric Clinics of North America, 21*(1), 119–133.
Kaufman, A. S., & Kaufman, N. L. (2004). *Kaufman Assessment Battery for children* (2nd ed.). Circle Pines, MN: American Guidance Service.
Kern, L., Hilt, A. M., & Gresham, F. (2004). An evaluation of the functional behavioral assessment process used with students with or at risk for emotional and behavioral disorders. *Education & Treatment of Children, 27*(4), 440–452.
Killu, K. (2008). Developing affective behavior intervention plans: Suggestions for school personnel. *Intervention in School and Clinic, 43*(3), 140–149.

Kilpatrick, D. A. (2014). *Essentials of assessing, preventing and overcoming reading difficulties.* Hoboken, NJ: John Wiley & Sons.

Kirby, J. R., Georgiou, G. K., Martinussem, R., & Parilla, R. (2010). Naming speed and reading: From prediction to instruction. *Reading Research Quarterly, 45,* 341–464.

Kisilevsky, B. S., Hains, S. M. J., Lee, K., Xie, X., Huang, H., Ye, H.-H., et al. (2003). Effects of experience on fetal voice recognition. *Psychological Science, 14,* 220–224.

Klassen, R. M., Tze, V. M. C., & Hannok, W. (2013). Internalizing problems of adults with learning disabilities: A meta-analysis. *Journal of Learning Disabilities, 46,* 317–327.

Kofler, M. J., Rapport, M. D., Bolden, J., Sarver, D. E., & Raiker, J. S. (2010). ADHD and working memory: The impact of central executive deficits and exceeding storage/rehearsal capacity on observed inattentive behavior. *Journal of Abnormal Child Psychology, 38,* 149–161.

Korkman, M., Kirk, U., & Kemp, S. (1998). *The NEPSY Manual.* San Antonio, TX: The Psychological Corporation.

Krawczyk, D. C., McClelland, M. M., Donovan, C. M., Tillman, G. D., & Maguire, M. J. (2010). An fMRI investigation of cognitive stages in reasoning by analogy. *Brain Research, 1342,* 63–73.

Ladd, G. W., & Burgess, K. B. (2001). Do relational risk and protective factors moderate the links between childhood aggression and early psychological and school adjustment? *Child Development, 72,* 1579–1601.

Landreth, G. L. (2002). Therapeutic limit setting in the play therapy relationship. *Professional Psychology: Research and Practice, 33*(6), 529–535.

Lang, L. (1997). Too much time out. *Teacher Magazine, 8,* 6–7.

Larson, R., Raffaella, M., Maryse, R., Ham, M., & Jewel, L. (1990). Ecology of depression in late childhood and early adolescence: A profile of daily states and activities. *Faculty Publications, Department of Psychology.* Paper 196. Lincoln, NE: University of Nebraska – Lincoln.

Law, J., & Garret, Z. (2004). Speech and language therapy: Its potential role in CHAMS. *Child and Adolescent Mental Health, 9*(2), 50–55.

LD Online (1999). Retrieved from ldonline.org/article.6313?theme=print.

Lee, M. (1989). When is an object not and object? The effect of "meaning" upon the copying of line drawings. *British Journal of Psychology, 80,* 15–37.

Leerkes, E. M., Paradise, M., O'Brien, M., Calkins, S. D., & Lange, G. (2008). Emotion and cognition processes in preschool children. *Merrill–Palmer Quarterly,* 54, 102–124.

Lemov, D. (2015). *Teach like a champion 2.0: 62 techniques that put students on the path to college.* San Francisco, CA: Jossey Boss.

Lezak, M. D. (1995). *Neuropsychological assessment* (3rd ed.). New York, NY: Oxford University Press.

Lim, C. Y., Tan, P. C., Koh, C., Koh, E., Guo, H., Ysoff, N. D., Tan, T. et al. (2015). Beery–Buktinica Developmental Test of Visual-Motor Integration (Beery-VMI): Lessons for exploration of cultural variations in visual-motor integration performance of preschoolers. *Child: Care, Health and Development, 41*(2), 213–221.

Liu, Jianghong (2004). Childhood externalizing behavior: Theory and implications. *Journal of Child and Adolescent Psychiatric Nursing, 17*(3), 93–103.

Lobier, M., Dubois, M., Valdois, S. (2013). The role of visual processing speed in reading speed development. *PLoS ONE, 8*(4), 1–10.

Lonigan, C. J., Bloomfield, B. G., Anthony, J. L., Bacon, K. D., Phillips, B. M., & Samwel, C. S. (1999). Relations among emergent literacy skills, behavior problems, and social competence in preschool children from low- and middle-income backgrounds. *Topics in Early Childhood Special Education, 19*(1), 40–53.

Lukowski, A. F., & Bauer, P. J. (2013). Long-term memory in infancy and early childhood. In P. J. Bauer and R. Fivush (Eds.), *The Wiley handbook on the development of children's memory, Vol. I/II* (pp. 230–254). Chichester: John Wiley & Sons.

Lum, J., Kidd, E., Davis, S., & Conti-Ramsden, G. (2010). Longitudinal study of declarative and procedural memory in primary school-aged children. *Australian Journal of Psychology, 62*, 139–148.

Luria, A. R. (1966). *Higher cortical functions in man.* New York, NY: Basic Books.

Maag, J. W. (2001). *Powerful struggles: Managing resistance, building rapport.* Longmont, CO: Sopris Press.

Maag, J. W. (2001). Rewarded by punishment: Reflections on the disuse of positive reinforcement in schools. *Exceptional Children, 67*, 173–186.

Maag, J. W., & Reid, R. (2006). Depression among students with learning disabilities: Assessing the risk. *Journal of Learning Disabilities, 39*, 3–10.

Main, M., & Solomon, J. (1986). Discovery of an insecure-disorganized/disoriented attachment pattern. In T. B. Brazelton & M. W. Yogman (Eds.), *Affective development in infancy.* Norwood, NJ: Ablex.

Margurussa, T. (2012, October). Tips for teaching high frequency words. *Scholastic News.* Retrieved from www.scholastic.com/teachers/top-teaching/2012/10/tips-teaching-high-frequency-and-sight-words.

Marr, D., Windsor, M., & Cermak, S. (2001). Handwriting readiness: Locatives and visuomotor skill in the kindergarten year. *Early Childhood Research and Practice, 34*(1), 1–28.

Martinovitch, J. (2005). *Creative expressive activities and Asperger's syndrome: Social and emotional skills and positive life goals for adolescents and young people.* Philadelphia, PA: Jessica Kingsley Publishers.

Mascolo, J. T., Alfonso, V. C., & Flanagan, D. P. (2014). *Essentials of planning, selecting, and tailoring interventions for unique learners.* Hoboken, NJ: John Wiley & Sons.

Mayer, D., Sodian, B., Koerber, S., & Schwippert, K. (2014). Scientific reasoning in elementary school children: Assessment and relations with cognitive abilities. *Learning and Instruction, 29*, 43–55.

McBride-Chang, C., & Kail, R. V. (2002). Cross-cultural similarities in the predictors of reading acquisition. *Child Development, 73*, 1392–1407.

McClelland, M. M., Cameron, C. E., Connor, C. M., Farris, C. L., Jewkes, A. M., & Morrison, F. J. (2007). Links between behavioral regulation and preschoolers' literacy, vocabulary, and math skills. *Developmental Psychology, 43*, 947–959.

McCloskey, G., Gilmartin, C., & Vitanza, B. S. (2014). Interventions for students with executive skills and executive functions difficulties. In J. T. Mascolo, V. C. Alfonso, & D. P. Flanagan (Eds.), *Essentials of planning, selecting and tailoring interventions for unique learners.* Hoboken, NJ: John Wiley & Sons.

McCutchen, D. (1996). A capacity theory of writing: Working memory in composition. *Educational Psychology Review, 8*, 299–325.

McHale, K., & Cermak, S. A. (1992). Fine motor activities in elementary school: Preliminary findings and provisional implications for children with fine motor problems. *American Journal of Occupational Therapy, 46*, 982–1001.

McNulty, R. J., & Gloeckler, L. C. (2011). *Fewer, clearer, higher Common Core State Standards: Implications for students receiving special education services.* Rexford, NY: International Center for Leadership in Education.

Meehan, B. T., Hughes, J. L., & Cavell T. A. (2003). Teacher–child relationships as compensatory resources for aggressive children. *Child Development, 74*, 1145–1157.

Mercier, T. (2014). Time out & teaching self-regulation. Retrieved from www.responsiveclassroom.org/time-out-teaching-self-regulation/.

Merriam-Webster. (2016). *Merriam-Webster's Dictionary of English Usage* (New Edition). Martinsburg, MV.

Miller, A. L., Seifer, R., Stroud, L., Sheinkopf, S. J., & Dickstein, S. (2006). Biobehavioral indices of emotion regulation relate to school attitudes, motivation, and behavior problems in a low-income preschool sample. *Annals of the New York Academy of Science, 1094*, 325–329.

Miller, C. A., Kail, R., Leonard, L. B., & Tomblin, J. B. (2001). Speed of processing in children with specific language impairment. *Journal of Speech, Language and Hearing Research, 44*, 416–433.

Miller, C. A., Leonard, L. B., Kail, R., Zhang, X., Tomblin, J. B., & Francis, D. J. (2006). Response time in 14-year-olds with language impairment. *Journal of Speech, Language and Hearing Research, 49*, 712–728.

Miller, J. A. (2010). Assessing and intervening with children and internalizing disorders. In D. C. Miller (Ed.), *Best practices in school neuropsychology: Guidelines for effective practice, assessment, and evidence-based intervention*. Hoboken, NJ: John Wiley & Sons.

Min Shim, J. (2014). Multicultural education as an emotional situation: Practice encountering the unexpected in teacher education. *Journal of Curriculum Studies, 24*(1), 116–137.

Minear, M., & Shah, P. (2006). Sources of working memory deficits in children and possibilities for remediation. In S. J. Pickering (Ed.), *Working memory and education*. Burlington, MA: Elsevier.

Misurell, J., Springer, C., Acosta, L., Liotta, L., & Kranzler, A. (2014). Game-based Cognitive-Behavioral Therapy individual model (GB-CBT-IM) for child sexual abuse: A preliminary outcome study. *Psychological Trauma: Theory, Research, Practice and Policy, 6*(3), 250–258.

Mocan, O., Stanciu, O., & Visu-Petra, L. (2014). Relating individual differences in internalizing symptoms to emotional attention set-shifting in children. *Anxiety, Stress & Coping: An International Journal, 27*(5), 509–526.

Morel, P., & Berzins, D. (2003). *Accommodations and strategies that work for me: A self-assessment inventory. LD Resource Guide*. Retrieved from www.disabilityissues.ca/english/index.html.

Morgan, P. L., Farka, G., Tufis, P. A., & Sperling, R. A. (2008). Are reading and behavior problems risk factors for each other? *Journal of Learning Disabilities, 41*(5), 417–436.

Morrison, A. B., & Chein, J. M. (2011). Does working memory training work? The promise and challenges of enhancing cognition by training working memory. *Psychonomic Bulletin Review, 18*, 46–60.

Mortimer, S., Adamsky, S., & McLaughlin, T. F. (1998). Use of isolated time out to reduce aggression and non-compliance with an elementary school student with severe behavior disorders: A long-term analysis. *International Journal of Special Education, 13*(1), 34–45.

Moss, E., Rousseau, D., Parent, S., St-Laurent, D., & Saintonge, J. (1998). Correlates of attachment at school age: Maternal reported stress, mother–child interaction, and behavior problems. *Child Development, 69*(5), 1390–1405.

Nanez, J. E., & Yonas, A. (1994). Effects of luminance and texture motion on infant defensive reactions to optical collision. *Infant Behavior and Development, 17*, 165–174.

Newhall, P. W. (2008). Teaching time management to students with learning disabilities. Adapted from *Study skills: research-based teaching strategies*. Prides Crossing, MA: Landmark School.

Nicolopoulou, A., & Ilgaz, H. (2013). What do we know about pretend play and narrative development? A response to Lillard, Lerner, Hopkins, Dore, Smith and Palquist on "The impact of pretend play on children's development: A review of the evidence." *American Journal of Play Therapy, 6*(1), 55–81.

Niles-Campbell, N., Tam, C., Mays, J., & Skidmore, G. (2008). Understanding the development of keyboarding skills in children with fine motor difficulties. *Occupational Therapy Now, 10*(4), 13–15.

Northey, W. F., Jr., Wells, K. C., Silverman, W. K., & Bailey, C. E. (2003). Childhood behavioral and emotional disorders. *Journal of Marital and Family Therapy, 29*, 523–545.

Numeroff, L. (1985). *If you give a mouse a cookie.* New York, NT: HarperCollins.

Numeroff, L. (1991). *If you give a moose a muffin.* New York, NY: HarperCollins.

Numeroff, L. (1998). *If you give a pig a pancake.* New York, NY: HarperCollins.

Numeroff, L. (2008). *If you give a cat a cupcake.* New York, NY: HarperCollins.

Oakes, L. M., & Luck, S. J. (2014). Short-term memory in infancy. In P. J. Bauer and R. Fivush (Eds.), *The Wiley handbook on the development of children's memory, Vol. I/II* (pp. 151–180). Chichester: John Wiley & Sons.

Ostrosky, M. M., Jung, E. Y., & Hemeter, M. L. (n.d.). Helping children make transitions between activities. Center on the Social and Emotional Foundations for Early Learning. Retrieved from http://csefel.vanderbilt.edu/resources/wwb/wwb4.html.

Otaiba, S. A., Wagner, R. K., & Miller, B. (2014). "Waiting to fail" redux: Understanding inadequate response to intervention. *Learning Disability Quarterly, 37*(3), 129–133.

Palumbo, D. R., & Diehl, J. (2007). Managing attentional disorders. In S. J. Hunger & J. Donders (Eds.), *Pediatric neuropsychological intervention.* New York, NY: Cambridge University Press.

Parisi, D. M., Ihlo, T., & Glover, T. A. (2014). Screening within a multitiered early prevention model: Using assessment to inform instruction and promote students' response to intervention. In R. J. Kettler, T. A. Glover, C. A. Albers, & K. A. Feeney-Kettler (Eds.), *Universal screening in educational settings: Evidence-based decision making for schools.* Washington, DC: American Psychological Association.

Parten, M. (1932). Social participation among preschool children. *Journal of Abnormal and Social Psychology, 27*(3), 243–269.

Pett, M. (2014). *The girl and the bicycle.* New York, NY: Simon & Schuster.

Phillips, L. H., Tunstall, M., & Channon, S. (2007). Exploring the role of working memory in dynamic social cue encoding using dual task methodology. *Journal of Nonverbal Behavior, 31*, 137–152.

Pichlas, T., Gracey, J., & Currie, K. (2006). *Teaching all students: Staff guide to accommodations and modifications.* Bad Axe and Ubly, MI: Huron Intermediate School District and Ubly Community Schools.

Pierucci, J. M., O'Brien, C. T., McInnis, M. A., Gilpin, A. T., & Barber, A. B. (2014). Fantasy-oriented constructs and related executive function development in preschool: Developmental benefits to executive functions by being a fantasy-oriented child. *International Journal of Behavioral Development, 38*, 62–69.

Pitchford, N. J., & Mullen, K. T. (2003). The development of conceptual colour categories in pre-school children: Influence of perceptual categorization. *Visual Cognition, 10*, 51–77.

Poll, G. H., Miller, C. A., Mainela-Arnold, E., Adams, K. D., Misra, M., & Park, J. S. (2013). Effects of children's working memory capacity and processing speed on their sentence imitation performance. *International Journal of Language & Communication Disorders, 48*(3), 329–342.

Posner, M. I., & Rothbart, M. K. (2007). *Educating the human brain.* Washington, DC: American Psychological Association.

Power-deFur, L. (2015). *Common core state standards and the speech-language pathologist: Standards-based intervention for special populations.* San Diego, CA: Plural Publishing.
Raskin, L. A., Maital, S., & Bornstein, M. H. (1983). Perceptual categorization of color: A life-span study. *Psychological Research*, 45, 639–649.
Raskinski, T. V. (2012). Why fluency should be hot! *The Reading Teacher*, *65*(1), 24–30.
Reinstein, D. K. (2006). *To hold and be held: The therapeutic school as a holding environment.* New York, NY: Routledge.
Reinstein, D. K., & Burau, D. E. (2014). *Integrating neuropsychological and psychological evaluations: Assessing and helping the whole child.* New York, NY: Routledge.
Reynolds, C. R., & Kamphaus, R. W. (2015). *The behavioral assessment system for children* (3rd ed.). Bloomington, MN: Pearson.
Riccio, C. A., Sullivan, F. R., & Cohen, M. J. (2010). *Neuropsychological assessment and intervention for childhood and adolescent disorders.* Hoboken, NJ: John Wiley & Sons.
Rief, S. F. (2005). *How to reach and teach children with ADD/ADHD: Practical techniques, strategies and interventions* (2nd ed.). San Francisco, CA: Jossey-Bass.
Riley, P. (2011). *Attachment theory and the teacher–student relationship: A practical guide for teachers, teacher educators and school leaders.* London: Routledge.
Riner, P. S., & Tanase, M. (2014). Inviting calm within: ADD, neurology and mindfulness. *Journal of Invitation Theory and Practice*, *20*, 11–25.
Robb, L. (2010). *Teaching reading in middle school: A strategic approach to teaching reading that improves comprehension and thinking* (2nd ed.). New York, NY: Scholastic.
Roediger, H. L. (1990). Implicit memory: Retention without remembering. *American Psychologist*, 45, 1043–1056.
Rogers, S. (2011). Play and pedagogy: A conflict of interests? In S. Rogers (Ed.), *Rethinking play and pedagogy in early childhood education: Concepts, contexts and cultures.* New York, NY: Routledge.
Roid, G. H. (2003). *Stanford-Binet intelligence scales, 5.* Rolling Meadows, IL: Riverside Publishing.
Romano, E., Babchishin, L., Pagani, L. S., & Kohen, D. (2010). School readiness and later achievement: Replication and extension using a nationwide Canadian survey. *Developmental Psychology*, 46, 995–1007.
Rosenblum, S., Weiss, P. L., & Parush, S. (2003). Product and process evaluation of handwriting difficulties. *Education Psychology Review*, *12*(1), 41–81.
Roskos, K. A., Patton, O. T., & Lenhart, L. A. (2004). *Oral language and literacy in preschool: Talk, reading and writing* (2nd ed.). Newark, DE: International Reading Association.
Ross-Sheehy, S., Oakes, L. M., & Luck, S. J. (2003). The development of visual short-term memory capacity in infants. *Child Development*, *74*(6), 1807–1822.
Rovee-Collier, C. (1999). The development of infant memory. *Current Directions in Psychological Science*, *8*(3), 80–85.
Rubin, K. H., Bukowski, W. M., & Parker, J. G. (2006). Peer interactions, relationships and groups. In W. Damon, R. M. Lerner, & N. Eisenberg (Eds.), *Handbook of child psychology Vol. 3* (6th ed.). New York, NY: Wiley Publishing.
Ruff, H. A., & Rothbart, M. K. (1996). *Attention in early development: Themes and variations.* New York, NY: Oxford University Press.
Rycus, J. S., & Hughes, R.C. (1998). *The field guide to child welfare, Vol. III: Child development and child welfare.* Washington, DC: Child Welfare League of America Press.
Saarni, C. (2000). *Encyclopedia on early child development: Emotions.* Child Encyclopedia.com.

Safer, D., Zito, J., & Fine, E. (1996). Increased methylphenidate usage for attention deficit hyperactivity disorder in the 1990's. *Pediatrics, 98*, 1084–1088.

Saffran, J. R., Werker, J. F., & Werner, L. A. (2006). The infant's auditory world: Hearing, speech, and the beginnings of language. In D. Kuhn & R. S. Siegler (Eds.), W. Damon (Series Ed.), *Handbook of child psychology: Vol. 2. Cognition, perception, and language* (6th ed., pp. 58–108). Hoboken, NJ: Wiley.

Safran, D. (2002). *Art therapy and AD/HD: Diagnostic and therapeutic approaches*. Philadelphia, PA: Jessica Kingsley Publishers.

Samuels, S. J., & Eisenberg, P. (1981). A framework for understanding the reading process. In F. J. Pirozzolo & M. C. Wittrock (Eds.), *Neuropsychological and cognitive processes in reading*. New York, NY: Academic Press.

Sasso, G. M., Conroy, M. A., Janine, P. S., & Fox, J. J. (2001). Slowing down the bandwagon: The misapplication of functional assessment for students with emotional or behavioral disorders. *Behavioral Disorders, 26*(4), 282.

Sattler, J. (2008). *Assessment of children: Cognitive foundations* (5th ed.). San Diego, CA: Jerome M. Sattler.

Sautter, E., & Wilson, K. (2016a). *Whole body listening Larry at home!* (2nd ed.). Santa Clara, CA: Social Thinking.

Sautter, E., & Wilson, K. (2016b). *Whole body listening Larry at school!* (2nd ed.). Santa Clara, CA: Social Thinking.

Scardamalia, M., Bereiter, C., & Goleman, H. (1982). The role of production factors in writing ability. In M. Nystrand (Ed.), *What writers know: The language process and structure of written discourse*. New York, NY: Academic Press, 173–210.

Scarry, R. (1981). *The gingerbread man*. New York, NY: Random House.

Schmuckler, M. A. (1997). Children's postural sway in response to low- and high-frequency visual information for oscillation. *Journal of Experimental Psychology: Human Perception and Performance, 23*(2), 528–545.

Schneider, W. (2010). Metacognition and memory development in childhood and adolescence. In H. S. Waters & W. Schneider (Eds.), *Metacognition, strategy use, and instruction* (pp. 54–84). New York, NY: Guilford Press.

Schneider, W. (2015). *Memory development from early childhood through emerging adulthood*. Cham, Switzerland: Springer.

Schneider, W., & Ornstein, P. (2015). The development of children's memory. *Child Development Perspectives, 9*(3), 190–195.

Schneider, W., & Pressley, M. (1997). *Memory development between two and twenty* (2nd ed.). Mahwah, NJ: Erlbaum.

Schrank, F. A., McGrew, K. S., & Mather, N. (2014). *Woodcock-Johnson IV tests of cognitive abilities*. Falling Meadows, IL: Riverside.

Scieszka, J., & Smith, L. (1992). *The stinky cheese man and other fairly stupid tales*. New York, NY: Viking Press.

Seaman, J. (2014). *Accommodations for cognitive and academic deficits: A compendium of accommodations and instructional strategies corresponding to the Woodcock-Johnson III Cognitive and Achievement clusters*. Granite Schools, UT.

Semrud-Clikeman, M., Kamphaus, R. W., Teeter, P. A., Vaughn, M. (1997). Assessment of behavior and personality in the neuropsychological diagnosis of children. In C. R. Reynolds & E. Fletcher-Janzen (Eds.), *Handbook of clinical child neuropsychology* (2nd ed.). New York, NY: Plenum Press.

Shah, N. (2011). Survey of school, district workers show wider use of RTI. *Education Week*. Retrieved from http://blogs.edweek.org/edweek/speced/2011/08/yet_another_study_shows_the.html.

Shannon, D. (1998). *No, David!* New York, NY: Blue Sky Press.
Shapiro, L. E. (2004). *101 ways to teach children social skills: A ready-to-use reproducible activity book*. Farmingville, NY: Lawrence Shapiro and the Bureau For At-Risk Youth.
Shields, A., Dickstein, S., Seifer, R., Giusti, L., Magee, K. D., & Spritz, B. (2001). Emotional competence and early school adjustment: A study of preschoolers at risk. *Early Education & Development*, 12, 73–96.
Silver, R. B., Measelle, J., Essex, M., & Armstrong, J. M. (2005). Trajectories of externalizing behavior problems in the classroom: Contributions of child characteristics, family characteristics, and the teacher–child relationship during the school transition. *Journal of School Psychology*, *43*, 39–60.
Slater, A., Morison, V., Town, C., & Rose, D. (1985). Movement perception and identity constancy in the new-born baby. *British Journal of Developmental Psychology*, *3*, 211–220.
Slobodkina, E. (1945). *Caps for sale: A tale of a peddler, some monkeys and their monkey business*. New York, NY: William R. Scott.
Smith, L. B. (2003). Learning to recognize objects. *Psychological Science*, *14*, 244–250.
Smith, S. R. (2007). Integrating neuropsychology and personality assessment with children and adolescents. In S. R. Smith & L. Handler (Eds.), *The clinical assessment of children and adolescents: A practitioner's handbook*. New York, NY: John Wiley & Sons.
Sobol, T. J., & Pianta, R. C. (2012). Recent trends in research on teacher-child relationships. *Attachment and Human Development*, *14*(3), 213–231.
Sprenger, M. (2005). *How to teach students to remember*. Alexandria, VA: Association for Supervision and Curriculum Development.
Squire, L. R. (1982). The neuropsychology of human memory. *Annual Review of Neuroscience*, *5*, 241–273.
Squire, L. R. (2004). Memory systems of the brain: A brief history and current perspective. *Neurobiology of Learning and Memory*, *82*, 171–177.
Stannard, L., Wolfgang, C. H., Jones, I., & Phelps, P. (2001). A longitudinal study of the predictive relations among construction play and mathematical achievement. *Early Child Development and Care*, *167*(1), 115–125.
Stephens, T. L. (2016). Understanding internalizing behaviors: Implications for students. *Review360Pearson*. Retrieved from www.pearsoned.com/education-blog/understanding-internalizing-behaviors-implications-for-students/.
Sugai, G., & Horner, R. (2006). A promising approach for expanding and sustaining the implementation of school wide positive behavior support. *School Psychology Review*, *35*, 245–259.
Sulkowski, M. L., Joyce, D. K., & Storch, E. A. (2011). Treating childhood anxiety in schools: Service delivery in a response to intervention paradigm. *Journal of Child Family Studies*, *21*, 938–947.
Szalavitz, M., & Perry, B. (2011). *Born for love*. New York, NY: Harper.
Taylor, S. J., Barker, L. A., Heavey, L. H., & McHale, S. (2013). The typical developmental trajectory of social and executive functions in late adolescence and early adulthood. *Developmental Psychology*, *49*(7), 1253–1265.
Teller, D. Y. (1998). Spatial and temporal aspects of infant color vision. *Vision Research*, *38*, 3275–3282.
Terban, M. (1983). *In a pickle and other funny idioms*. New York, NY: Houghton Mifflin.
Thibodeau, R. B., Gilpin, A. T., Brown, M. M., & Meyer, B. A. (2016). The effects of fantastical pretend-play on executive functions: An intervention study. *Journal of Experimental Child Psychology*, *145*, 120–138.

Thompson, S. (1998). Developing an instructional plan for the student with NLD. *LD Online*. Retrieved from www.ldonline.org/article/.

Tigner, R. B. (1999). Putting memory research to good use. *College Teaching*, *47*(4), 149.

Todd, A. W., Horner, R. H., Vanater, S. M., & Schneider, C. F. (1997). Working together to make change: An example of positive behavioral support for a student with traumatic brain injury. *Education and Treatment of Children*, *20*, 425–440.

Tramontana, M. G., & Hooper, S. R. (1997). Neuropsychology of child psychopathology. In C. R. Reynolds & E. Fletcher-Janzen (Eds.), *Handbook of clinical child neuropsychology* (2nd ed.). New York, NY: Plenum Press Corporation.

Trentacosta, C. J., & Izard, C. E. (2007). Kindergarten children's emotion competence as a predictor of their academic competence in first grade. *Emotion*, *7*, 77–88.

Truesdale, S. P. (1990). Whole-body listening: Developing active auditory skills. *Language, Speech, and Hearing Services in Schools*, *21*, 183–184.

Uberti, H. Z., Mastropieri, M. A., & Scruggs, T. E. (2004). Check it off: Individualizing a math algorithm for students with disabilities via self-monitory checklists. *Intervention in School and Clinic*, *39*(5), 269–275.

U.S. Department of Education (2004). *Individuals with Disabilities Education Act* (34 CFR §300.34). Washington, DC: U.S. Government Printing Office.

van der Kolk, B. (1994). The body keeps the score: Memory and the evolving psychobiology of post-traumatic stress. *Harvard Reviews in Psychiatry*, *1*, 253–265.

van der Kolk, B. (2014). *The body keeps the score: Brain, mind and body in the healing of trauma*. New York, NY: Viking Press.

Vennum, A., & Vennum, D. (2013). Expanding our reach: Marriage and family therapists in the public school system. *Contemporary Family Therapy*, *35*, 41–58.

Verdine, B. N., Golinkoff, R. M., Hirsh-Pasek, K., Newcombe, N. S., Filipowicz, A. T., & Chang, A. (2013). Deconstructing building blocks: Preschoolers' spatial assembly performance relates to early mathematical skills. *Child Development*, 1–15.

Verschueren, K. (2015). Middle childhood teacher–child relationships: Insights from an attachment perspective and remaining challenges. In G. Bosmans & K. A. Kerns (Eds.), *Attachment in middle childhood: Theoretical advances and new directions in an emerging field: New Directions for Child and Adolescent Development*, *148*, 77–91.

von Hofsten, C. (1974). Proximal velocity change as a determinant of space perception. *Perception & Psychophysics*, *15*(3), 488–494.

Vygotsky, L. (1978). Play and its role in the mental development of the child. *Soviet Psychology*, *5*(6), 6–18.

Waguespack, A., Vaccaro, T., & Continere, L. (2006). Functional behavioral assessment and intervention with emotional/behaviorally disordered students: In pursuit of state of the art. *International Journal of Behavioral Consultation & Therapy*, *2*(4), 463–474.

Wechsler, D. (2008). *Wechsler adult intelligence scale* (4th ed.). San Antonio, TX: The Psychological Corporation.

Wechsler, D. (2014). *Wechsler intelligence scale for children* (5th ed.). San Antonio, TX: The Psychological Corporation.

Wechsler, D. (2014). *Wechsler preschool and primary scale of intelligence* (4th ed.). San Antonio, TX: The Psychological Corporation.

Wilczenski, F., Konstam, V., Ferraro, B., & Kaplan, L. (2001). *School and classroom organizations affecting social and emotional learning outcomes.* U.S. Department of Education Educational Resources Information Center.

Williams, H. C., Conway, M. A., & Cohen, G. (2008). Autobiographical memory. In G. Cohen & M. A. Conway (Eds.), *Memory in the real world* (3rd ed.). Hove: Psychology Press.

Willner, C. J., Gatske-Kopp, L. M., & Bray, B. C. (2016). The dynamics of internalizing and externalizing comorbidity across the early school years. *Development and Psychopathology*, *28*(41), 1033–1052.

Winnicott, D. W. (1965). *The maturational processes and the facilitating environment*. London: Hogarth Press.

Winnicott, D. (1974). *Playing and reality*. Middlesex: Pelican Books.

Wolf, M. (2008). *Proust and the squid: The story and science of the reading brain*. Cambridge: Icon Books.

Wolf, M., & Bowers, P. G. (1999). The double-deficit hypothesis for the developmental dyslexias. *Journal of Educational Psychology*, *91*, 415–438.

Wolf, T. L., McLaughlin, T. F., & Williams, R. L. (2006). Time-out interventions and strategies: A brief review and recommendations. *International Journal of Special Education*, *21*(3), 22–29.

Wong, H. K., Wong, R. T., Jondahl, S. F., & Ferguson, O. F. (2014). *The classroom management book*. Mountain View, CA: Harry K. Wong.

Woolley, J. D., & Tullos, A. (2008). Imagination and fantasy. In M. Haith & J. Benson (Eds.), *Encyclopedia of infant and early childhood development* (pp. 117–127). Oxford: Elsevier.

Wu, S. S., Willcutt, E. G., Escovar, E., & Menon, V. (2014). Mathematics achievement and anxiety and their relation to internalizing and externalizing behaviors. *Journal of Learning Disabilities*, *47*(6), 503–514.

Ylvisaker, M., & Feeney, T. (2002). Executive functions, self-regulation, and learned optimism in pediatric rehabilitation: A review and implication for intervention. *Pediatric Rehabilitation*, *5*(2), 51–70.

Yonas, A., Arterberry, M. E., & Granrud, C. E. (1987). Four-month-old infants' sensitivity to binocular and kinetic information for three-dimensional object shape. *Child Development*, *58*, 910–971.

Yoshida, W., Dziobek, I., Kliemann, D., Heekeren, H. R., Friston, K. J., & Dlona, R. J. (2010). Cooperation and heterogeneity of the autistic mind. *Journal of Neuroscience*, *30*, 8815–8818.

Zeigler Dendy, C. A. (2011). *Teaching teens with ADD, ADHD and executive functions deficits: A quick reference guide for teachers and parents* (2nd ed.). Bethesda, MD: Woodbine House.

Index

For Product Safety Concerns and Information please contact our EU representative GPSR@taylorandfrancis.com Taylor & Francis Verlag GmbH, Kaufingerstraße 24, 80331 München, Germany

Batch number: 10753468

Printed by Printforce, the Netherlands